High-Reliability
HEALTHCARE

High-Reliability
HEALTHCARE

IMPROVING
PATIENT SAFETY
AND
OUTCOMES
WITH
SIX SIGMA

SECOND EDITION

Robert Barry ◆ Amy C. Smith
Clifford E. Brubaker

ACHE Management Series

Acquisitions editor: Janet Davis; Project manager: Andrew Baumann; Manuscript editor: Adin Bookbinder; Cover designer: Brad Norr; Layout: PerfecType

Health Administration Press
A division of the Foundation of the American
    College of Healthcare Executives
One North Franklin Street, Suite 1700
Chicago, IL 60606-3529
(312) 424-2800

Contents

Preface

*Since the first edition was published in 2002, the healthcare industry
has taken a keen interest in High-Reliability Organizations, driven
by the desire to improve patient safety. This is to be commended.*

SIX SIGMA IS complementary to the High-Reliability Organization culture, providing a tool kit for reducing error, understanding variability, and managing change. Six Sigma as a stepping stone to the High-Reliability Healthcare Organization has been recognized by Chassin and Loeb (2013), writing for The Joint Commission.

This second edition explains how Six Sigma fits into and complements the High-Reliability Organization. This edition expands on Lean operations to include scheduling with and without queuing, with additional cases added to the set. This edition also addresses

- interruptions and how to design workflow, given that interruptions are not going to go away;
- communications using Six Sigma rules; and
- computerization, including what to consider when adapting computerization and the difficulties that computers entail.

The additional material on the Health Administration Press website is updated and includes worksheets for the new cases.

Robert Barry, PhD
Amy C. Smith, DNP, FACHE
Clifford E. Brubaker, PhD

Companion Website

This book is accompanied by a website—www.ache.org/books/6Sigma—that includes the lists of data required to work the cases to spare the reader from having to rekey all the data. The website also contains sample spreadsheets showing the application of the statistical functions used in the book. A few of the cases are also worked in full on the website to show the application of the method being taught.

The following are on the website:

1. Data for all cases in Microsoft Excel 2016 format
2. Complete solutions for indicative cases
3. PowerPoint templates for case reports
4. Complete analysis of examples not carried to completion in the text
5. A Microsoft Excel icebreaker

Instructor Resources

This book is accompanied by an Instructor's Manual. This Instructor's Manual includes lectures for 15 three-hour class sessions, discussion topics, assignments, supplementary papers, and PowerPoint slides. The Instructor's Manual can also be used for executive short courses and on-site consultations.

For the most up-to-date information about this book and its Instructor Resources, go to www.ache.org/HAP and browse for the book's title or author name.

This book's Instructor Resources are available to instructors who adopt this book for use in their course. For access information, please e-mail hapbooks@ache.org.

Acknowledgments

THE AUTHORS ARE pleased to acknowledge Matthew R. Barry, PhD, of Houston, Texas, for many helpful discussions and for his assistance with the preparation of this book. The authors are also pleased to acknowledge the attentive and enlightened work of copy editor Adin Bookbinder.

Patient Safety, High-Reliability Organizations, and Six Sigma

Every organization has a culture.

THE AIRCRAFT CARRIER is months behind its construction schedule, with problems everywhere. An admiral is assigned to straighten things out. On the first day, the admiral enters the Monday morning production meeting, picks up the two-inch-thick computer report on late items, turns to the last item on the last page, and opens the meeting by saying, "Good morning. Who can tell me about this cotter pin?" (US Navy Commander 1974).

"Yes, Admiral, but we really need your help with the propeller warp. That's what's killing the schedule."

"Yes, thank you, we'll get to that. Right now I want to know about this cotter pin."

"Yes, Admiral, but our practice has been to focus on the key items on the critical path."

"Yes, yes. Now who can tell me about this cotter pin?"

Lots of squirming in chairs around the room. The next week, the late-items report was a few pages thinner. The second week, many more. By the end of the month, the late-items report was one page long, and that one page listed matters that were worthy of management attention, including the propeller warp. The other matters seemed to have taken care of themselves.

In a few meetings and with very few words, the new admiral had changed the culture from Management by Crisis to Taking Care of Little Things so They Won't Become Big Things.

Every organization embodies the culture that its CEO wants. Indeed, setting the culture is an important responsibility of the CEO. What culture does the CEO

1

want for the organization? Once the CEO decides and communicates the message, the organization, in its own interest, will respond and try to conform. Even organizations as complicated as today's healthcare organizations will respond.

Today's healthcare issues are patient safety and outcomes. With those in mind, many CEOs are looking to the High-Reliability Organization initiative, which studies other industries that execute high-stress and high-risk operations every day and have learned to succeed both in safety and in outcomes. Perhaps healthcare organizations can adapt lessons to the high-stress, thinly staffed, highly variable, often interrupted, partly computerized healthcare system of today.

It's worth a try.

Six Sigma provides a tool kit to help things along.

HIGH-RELIABILITY ORGANIZATIONS

Karl E. Weick and Kathleen M. Sutcliffe published the first edition of *Managing the Unexpected: Resilient Performance in an Age of Uncertainty* in 2001, laying the foundation for learning from organizations outside of healthcare that operate in trying conditions and yet manage to have few untoward events. The High-Reliability Organizations usually cited are the US Navy, the civilian nuclear power industry, and commercial aviation.

Weick and Sutcliffe conclude that these organizations all have developed a culture, from top management on down, that is essential to success:

- ◆ Anticipate—stay out of trouble.
- ◆ Contain—get out of trouble.

Note that "tolerate a certain amount of trouble" is not on the list.

To get results, management creates a culture with these characteristics:

- ◆ Anticipation
  - – Preoccupation with failure
  - – Sensitivity to operations
  - – Reluctance to simplify
- ◆ Containment
  - – Commitment to resilience
  - – Deference to expertise

These are cultural, attitudinal characteristics that can only exist by flowing from top management on down. The mechanics of designing tasks, establishing communications protocols, and so on, are left to middle managers and the professionals who operate within this culture.

An important feature in the culture of High-Reliability Organizations is the commitment to study near-misses as intently as studying events with untoward outcomes. The near-miss is more than twice as rich a learning opportunity as the event with an untoward outcome.

On the front end, the people involved are apt to be a little more forthcoming on what actually happened.

On the back end, something *good* happened. What? Who? When? Are there lessons that can be extracted and taught to others? Is something to be learned about equipment, about policy? Why did this solution work, and how did it come about?

For the event with an untoward outcome, studies will produce recommendations for change that are, at first, conjectural. Trials would be required to test out recommended changes. For the near-miss, one solution is already in hand, no conjecture required. Knowing there is at least one solution is a great advance in knowledge. Perhaps better solutions can be conjectured and tested; in the meantime, the one known solution can be put to use.

Going further with High-Reliability Organizations is beyond the scope of this present text. There are excellent sources elsewhere. In addition to the Weick and Sutcliffe book (2001), helpful information can be found online at www.high-reliability.org.

SIX SIGMA IN THE HIGH-RELIABILITY ORGANIZATION

Six Sigma is the culmination of a hundred years of learning about the management of people to get work done safely, promptly, and productively. If the terms *scientific management* and *statistical process control* were in vogue, then Six Sigma would be the latest embodiment of them. But Six Sigma is not stopwatches and clipboards.

Six Sigma is a way of thinking about tasks, thinking about multistep processes, thinking about people who work. Six Sigma is a way of teaching people to *do* that thinking. What is a properly designed task? How does Person A know that Person B received and understood a message? How does a system know if things are working or not? How can changes be made in an orderly and abiding way?

Six Sigma strives to reduce variability both by reducing error and by standardizing processes. The point of reducing variability is to make it possible to observe when the process is changing, to spot unusually good results to be learned from, and to spot unusually bad results so that the process can be corrected. The more avoidable variability is reduced, the earlier changes can be observed and acted on.

Six Sigma complements the High-Reliability Organization culture. Six Sigma observes and learns. Six Sigma contains. Six Sigma attends to the human factors of operations and change.

In healthcare, Six Sigma takes cognizance of the thin staffing, the interruptions, the complex communications, and the multi-shift and multidepartment care requirements—all factors that do not much occur in the High-Reliability Organizations referenced earlier.

Six Sigma for healthcare also takes cognizance of the still-immature computerization and rapid technology change now happening. The referenced High-Reliability Organizations are two or three generations ahead of healthcare in terms of computerization and can teach some lessons. However, some issues, particularly those dealing with human factors, are not entirely resolved, even in High-Reliability Organizations.

This book addresses the role and the substance of Six Sigma for existing healthcare organizations, supporting their adoption of the High-Reliability culture.

Mark R. Chassin and Jerod M. Loeb (2013, 461), writing for The Joint Commission, ask, "What can high-reliability organizations teach health care?" Chassin and Loeb laud the goal and then identify the ways today's hospitals do not match up with the ways High-Reliability Organizations achieve nearly error-free operations. Chassin and Loeb then assert that the way forward for the next several years is to focus on process improvement tools, specifically Lean, Six Sigma, and Change Management. This book covers all three.

Patient safety and patient care will benefit from Six Sigma and from the High-Reliability culture, both in the short run and the long run.

PATIENT SAFETY AND THE NEVER EVENTS

Ken Kizer, MD, introduced the term *Never Event* (AHRQ 2016) to label serious medical events that should *simply never occur* because the ways to prevent their occurrence are known. However, for some of them, particularly patient falls, there is no practical solution at the time of this writing.

Dr. Kizer introduced the following seven categories of Never Events in 2011 (AHRQ 2016):

1. *Surgical events*, such as a procedure performed on the wrong body part or patient or the retention of a foreign object in a patient after a procedure
2. *Product or device events*, such as a death or serious injury associated with the use of a contaminated drug or faulty device

3. *Patient protection events*, such as an incident of patient self-harm in a healthcare facility or the discharge or disappearance of a patient who is unable to make decisions alone
4. *Care management events*, including death or serious injury associated with a medication error, a fall, a severe pressure ulcer, the unsafe administration of blood products, or the failure to follow up on test results
5. *Environmental events*, such as a patient or staff death or injury associated with an electric shock, a burn, the use of bed rails, or the improper administration of oxygen or another gas while in a healthcare setting
6. *Radiologic events*, referring to a patient's or staff member's death or injury associated with the presence of a metal object in the magnetic resonance imaging area
7. *Criminal events*, such as the assault or abuse of a patient or staff member in a healthcare setting, the abduction of a patient, or an episode of care that is ordered or administered by an individual impersonating a licensed healthcare provider

The full list of Never Events is available at https://psnet.ahrq.gov/primers/primer/3/never-events. While several of them appear to be cotter pins, and somebody (probably several somebodies) should have been paying attention, there are exceptions. For instance, the incidence of patient falls has not improved much in recent years and stays around three or more per thousand bed days. That's three or four falls per week in a hundred-bed hospital. Thankfully, most are not fatal, but every fall puts a patient at serious risk. The point here is that no one knows how to do any better, despite large sums of money spent on alarms and gadgets. A good idea, a breakthrough, would be welcome.

Six Sigma deals with inadvertent error. Six Sigma has nothing to contribute to the prevention of malicious acts, such as those at the bottom of the list above. Those are important, but their solutions will have to be found elsewhere.

Word for the Day

Gossypiboma is the term for a sponge or towel retained in the body after surgery. This word comes from the Latin word for cotton, *gossypium*, combined with the Swahili word for place of concealment, *boma*.

Six Sigma

Six Sigma management methods set quantitative error rate objectives because experience has shown that, lacking specific goals, improvement is too slow and unsatisfactory for the needs of the day.

Six Sigma addresses error prevention, variability reduction, problem detection, problem solving, and managed change.

Six Sigma uses a collection of management practices to achieve its specified goal. Some of these practices are based on statistics, but many are not.

WHY SIX SIGMA?

You are a healthcare executive, or you expect to be one in due course. Your organization provides error-free care to your patients, your patients are discharged on schedule every time, every patient leaves with a correct financial statement and the proper instructions for at-home care, and you surely have attained peace of mind with regard to the management of your organization. Your facility has happy and loyal clientele, your staff has professional satisfaction, and your managers and resources are applied to positive purposes. If this describes your situation, you can close the book now with our congratulations.

If you have not quite reached that level of perfection but errors at your organization are exceedingly rare, you, too, can close the book now with our congratulations.

If you are still reading, this book may be what you've been looking for. You are committed voluntarily to the standards of The Joint Commission. This includes their standards for sentinel events: events that are life threatening or worse and for which a root-cause analysis and system-rectification plan are required. Six Sigma provides a systematic method for doing the analysis and rectifying the system.

You are committed to The Joint Commission standards for performance improvement. Six Sigma provides a systematic method for quantifying the existing system, defining trials, measuring progress, and characterizing long-term conformance.

You probably have a total quality management program, a continuous quality improvement program, and a quality assurance program, and you conform to the standard practices of each of your health professions. You undertook all of these as a means to an end: error-free provision of healthcare services.

You know instinctively the following:

◆ An organization that never makes errors has happy and loyal clientele.
◆ An organization that never makes errors is easy to manage.
◆ An organization that never makes errors has positive uses for resources.
◆ An organization that never makes errors attracts the best candidates for employment.
◆ An organization that never makes errors has peace of mind in the executive suite.

You also know that untoward events can happen, even in the best of organizations; therefore, you would wish to have at hand an organized management method for dealing with such events. Six Sigma provides such a method as it may be applied to products and services.

Efforts to improve production processes started in a systematic way before World War I with Taylor (1911), Gilbreth (1912), and others, who were known as efficiency experts. After World War I, a theory was developed that allowed the benefits to be applied systematically to all kinds of production. The best-known work was done by the telephone company at Bell Labs and in AT&T's manufacturing arm, known in those days as Western Electric. Other major companies did similar work; the AT&T work is best known because, having no competitors, AT&T did not mind publishing its findings. This body of work came to be called *scientific management.*

Frank Gilbreth, the efficiency expert, broke tasks down into small elements such as grasp, lift, and twist. He called these *therbligs,* derived from Gilbreth spelled backward. Gilbreth was played by Clifton Webb in the movie *Cheaper by the Dozen.*

Then came World War II. For three years, the American War Production Board ran the biggest command economy in the history of the world. Much of the production was done by giant companies that already knew scientific management, but much was also done by others who had been running small companies and who suddenly found themselves employing thousands of workers. These small companies needed help. The War Production Board saw to it that they got that help by mandating scientific management across the board. The results impressed our enemies and our allies alike as war material flowed from factories deprived of the 15 million men then in uniform and staffed instead by women, youngsters, oldsters, and just about everyone else who was available, few of whom had ever seen the inside of a factory before.

After the war, things returned to normal in the United States, with pent-up consumer demand replacing military demand in most industries. Without the War Production Board to tell them how to manage their work, some companies continued to apply scientific management, and some did not. With demand so high, not much discipline came from the marketplace to force manufacturers to perform well.

Meanwhile, General Douglas MacArthur saw the need to revive Japanese industry to get Japan's postwar economy going. The American market for manufactured goods was, relatively speaking, open to imports. Exporting to the United States would earn Japan some hard currency. Adding technology in the form of scientific management would speed things up, so MacArthur engaged a group of production experts from the United States to advise Japanese industrialists on how to manage production. Among these were two Americans who figure prominently in the story: C. Edwards Deming (Walton 1990) and Joseph M. Juran (1995). Both enjoyed long professional lives and advised Japanese clients for decades while maintaining their American practices.

Deming's 14 Steps

1. Create consistency of purpose.
2. Adopt the new philosophy.
3. Cease dependence on inspection.
4. End the practice of awarding business on the basis of price alone.
5. Improve constantly.
6. Institute training/retraining on the job.
7. Institute leadership for system improvement.
8. Drive out fear.
9. Break down barriers between departments.
10. Eliminate arbitrary quotas and slogans without providing resources.
11. Eliminate work standards (quotas) for management.
12. Remove barriers to pride of workmanship.
13. Institute education and self-improvement for everyone.
14. Transform everyone's job to transform the organization.

At the time, Japan had two big hurdles to overcome to implement a successful export strategy: It had no money, and it was a long way from the American market. Because of the lack of money, each raw material item was precious, and nothing could be wasted. Because of the country's distance from the American market, the Japanese manufacturers had to ship a product that would satisfy the American customer immediately on delivery because goods could not be shipped back to the factory to fix mistakes.

In short, the postwar Japanese companies had to build the product right, with no waste, or else their strategy would fail. Inspired by clear thinking on the matter and lacking any alternative, the Japanese exporters bore down and applied everything they could learn about low-error, low-loss manufacturing methods. They absorbed everything Deming and Juran had to offer, and they applied what they learned with zeal.

The Japanese started with transistor radios and motor scooters and moved over time to automobiles, sophisticated consumer products, computers, and capital goods, staying with the manufacturing discipline well after they had plenty of hard currency in the bank. The Japanese were discovering that their quality reputation earned them market share while minimizing costs.

This brings us up to the 1970s, which was a time of turmoil, stagflation, and malaise in the United States. American production was in such disarray that these popular-literature business theories emerged:

- Murphy's Law (Murphy 1949)—Anything that can go wrong will go wrong
- Parkinson's Law (Parkinson 1957)—Work expands to fill the time available
- The Peter Principle (Peter 1979)—Managers are promoted to their level of incompetence

American companies lost market share at home and abroad. The American government tried to help by imposing guidance in the form of quality assurance requirements on various civilian industries. These became institutionalized—that is, bureaucratized—over time, and they may or may not have been very helpful. American industrialists then trooped to Japan to learn from the quality masters.

In the 1980s, manufacturing started to turn around in the United States. Philip Crosby, head of quality assurance for the then-huge ITT corporation, had published a bestseller called *Quality Is Free* in 1979. Crosby observed (and it was confirmed by a great number of industries) that American companies were spending 20 percent of their time, capital, and management resources fixing things. If a fraction of that effort were put into doing something right in the first place, the company would recoup a lot of time and money.

Business rediscovered Deming and Juran. The *In Search of Excellence* books (Peters and Waterman 1982) sold by the carload. Companies signed up for total quality management and later for continuous quality improvement programs.

The American government created the Malcolm Baldrige Award to recognize efforts in the improvement of quality. The government later added a separate Baldrige Award for healthcare (NIST 2001). The International Organization of Standardization recognized quality assurance by issuing the ISO 9000 family of standards.

By 1990, American manufacturing companies were generally competent at producing quality goods and were holding their own. That did not, however, prove to be the end of the story. Motorola was the first to say that not enough progress was being made and that something more had to be done. If not, the quality level would never get to the standard they felt they *had* to meet to compete in their markets against very serious international competition. Motorola instituted the first Six Sigma program. Other major companies, most notably General Electric, IBM, and Texas Instruments, followed. These were followed in turn, curiously enough, by the Japanese company Sony. Transaction-oriented service companies such as American Express also took up Six Sigma practices; many banks are now following American Express's lead.

Crosby's 14 Points

1. Management commitment
2. Quality improvement team
3. Quality measurement
4. Cost-of-quality evaluation
5. Quality awareness
6. Corrective action
7. Ad-hoc committee for zero-defect planning
8. Supervisory training
9. Zero-defects day
10. Goal setting
11. Error-cause removal
12. Recognition
13. Quality councils
14. Do it over again

These companies had not been asleep between World War I and 1990; they had been leaders every step along the way. They had quality assurance programs, total quality management programs, and continuous quality improvement programs. They knew everything that could be known about scientific management. They were, as they had always been, leaders in production management.

So why did major companies decide they needed something new? Something more?

These leaders came to believe that maintaining their good management practices would result in products with a few defects per thousand. They wanted not to get to zero defects, because that would be impossible, but to a few defects per *million*; that is a thousand times better than what they had been doing, and they felt they had to get to that level. On the basis of their experience, they realized their existing programs would take a very long time—too long—to get where they wanted to be, and they did not have much time. They needed to take action.

Thus, Six Sigma. Six Sigma goes beyond "continuous improvement" programs to specific, numeric goals. These goals have now been shown to be attainable in many industries.

The Japanese experience is helpful because, in one human generation, postwar Japanese industry went through four complete technology generations—from handwork to hand-fed machines to self-feeding machines to self-controlling and self-monitoring machines. Most Japanese manufacturing was done in small batches, so special attention was paid to reducing setup time and understanding the flow of work.

Where is healthcare today? We are still doing a lot of handwork. Some mechanization and some computerization of instrumentation have arrived, and some robots are used—for example, in hip surgery. More mechanization is probably coming, but right now healthcare is largely handwork.

The contributions made back in the handwork stage of industrialization reduced back-breaking physical effort, organized the work and the tool crib, designed new tools, broke down tasks so they could be improved step by step, and taught workers to inspect their own work.

Many of these improvements were made specifically to reduce the frequency of worker error. With some thought, those lessons learned can today be applied to healthcare.

WHAT IS SIX SIGMA?

Six Sigma is a systematic method for improving the output of the organization by improving the quality of the system. This is done by reducing variability, preventing error, solving problems, managing change, and monitoring long-term performance in quantitative terms so that any incipient problems are detected before they become bothersome. Six Sigma is a quantitative method that deals with measures commonly called *quality measures*. Before discussing the application of a quality measure, having a definition of *quality* will be helpful.

The Institute of Medicine (IOM 2001, 1) defines quality as "the degree to which health services for individuals and populations increase the likelihood of desired health outcomes and are consistent with current professional knowledge." This goes in a good direction and would be hard to contradict but does not apply to something that can be quantified.

Crosby (1979, 15) provides an operable definition of quality by saying, "Quality is conformance to requirements." Nothing more, nothing less. This is a functional measure, and it works with something that can be quantified. Does the work meet the requirements or not? Does it pass or fail? What is the percentage of passes and the percentage of failures? No credit is given for being close or for good intentions; there is no extra credit for doing more than the specification required.

If the Crosby meaning of quality applies, what, then, is an error? To be consistent with Crosby, an error must be that which reduces conformance to requirements. An error need not, by itself, cause conformance to fail; an error need only detract.

In industry, a defective part is reworked or tossed in the reject pile. In healthcare, there is no reject pile, so any error causes rework, and rework takes time and resources.

Errors in healthcare service include the following:

- Administrative error in admission
- Incorrect or untimely diagnosis
- Error in medication
- Error in therapy or other treatment
- Administrative error in the patient record
- Untimely treatment
- Departure from nursing standard
- Departure from any other professional standard
- Error in prerelease patient indoctrination
- Administrative error in discharge
- Error in any financial statement
- Error in take-home instructions or medication
- Delayed discharge or too-soon readmission
- Other such action or inaction that has an effect on the timely treatment and discharge of the patient

Errors include direct injuries to the patient and all of the other things that detract from timely and effective treatment: a patient falls in the bathroom; an immobile patient is not turned in bed and risks pressure ulcers; X-rays are misfiled; supplies run out; schedules are botched; a department runs out of nurses and has to oblige some nurses to work a double shift; one department smooths out its workload by bunching up the work in the next department; billing errors are made. All these possibilities and many more detract from the organization's service to the patient and community.

Plenty of other management issues are not directly involved in service: unauthorized people parking in the doctors' parking spots; the capital budget campaign;

noisy helicopters annoying the neighbors; succession planning; recruiting. Six Sigma has nothing to offer for these topics.

SIX SIGMA AND QUALITY MANAGEMENT PROGRAMS

Baldrige Award for Health Care

The Baldrige Award is an annual recognition of performance quality, sponsored by the federal government's National Institute of Standards and Technology, the erstwhile Bureau of Standards. The Baldrige competition has been run for more than 25 years, and winning is a big feather in a cap. While the criteria vary slightly from year to year and are published annually, the main goal remains to boost awareness of and involvement in performance initiatives. Those pursuing the award may bemoan all the tracking charts. But because the Baldrige competition rewards improvement more than actual achievement, an organization that had been doing poorly and moves up to pretty good will score well and probably better than an organization that has been at the pinnacle of performance for years. There is merit in this approach, as the aim is to get lots of organizations to do better, while the top few continue to take care of themselves (NIST 2016).

Baldrige awards are given by sector. One of the sectors is healthcare.

The Balanced Score Card

The Balanced Score Card model for strategic management helps senior managers teach middle and junior managers to overcome the tendency to get caught up in the urgent matter of the day and pay some attention to important strategic interests. Applied to healthcare, the idea is to require all levels of management to report on four strategic topics, such as patient safety, nurse staffing, market share, and cost. One important contribution of the Balanced Score Card is to make all middle managers aware that they have a contribution to make to each of the key topics (Kaplan 2010; Research Gate 2016).

Total Quality Management

Total Quality Management, often called *TQM* (ASQ Quality Press 2013), attempts to adapt and apply to healthcare the concept of continuous improvement used in other industries. TQM may be seen as a forerunner of the current High-Reliability Organization initiatives, because effective TQM requires involvement of all levels of management, buy-in by professionals and other employees, and measures of performance.

The challenge with TQM is that continuous change in operations might be fine at the local level but self-defeating at higher levels of aggregation, by rewarding local optimization rather than global optimization. The Six Sigma approach is to standardize and then make a few discrete, larger changes that can be tested and measured globally.

HOW IS SIX SIGMA APPLIED?

Mature Six Sigma organizations simply include Six Sigma methods in everything they do, so no special attention is required. Before reaching that level of maturity, organizations select projects for Six Sigma attention, execute those projects, measure the results, and then take up more projects.

A Six Sigma project addresses work to be redesigned, a problem to be solved, a change to be instituted, or a key process or set of processes to be monitored so that any problem can be detected and resolved. Usually these three are connected; once a problem is solved, some change will be instituted to provide the solution, and the new process will be monitored over the long term to detect any new problems. Six Sigma error-prevention techniques will be implemented in the design of the solution to the problem.

Six Sigma projects are designed by black belts, who also oversee the projects. The projects are normally carried out by green belts. For early projects and major projects, the organization will assign a senior manager to act as a sponsor.

Some organizations have Six Sigma champions who promote Six Sigma; whether that is a good idea depends on the organization's culture. If the organization relies on the line organization to manage new methods, no particular need exists to also have champions. If the organization likes matrix management methods, champions may well fit in and accelerate the inculcation of Six Sigma into the organization as a whole.

To start, an organization needs two or three black belts and a few green belts. Theoretically, one black belt would be enough, but one is a fragile number. Black

Six Sigma Belts

- Green belts can carry out projects.
- Black belts can design and direct projects.
- Master black belts can train others and direct multiple projects.

belts are members of the organization who have an interest and are willing to accept training in something new; they do not have to have an advanced math background. Training can be done on-site or at a training facility, preferably by a Six Sigma training firm that specializes in healthcare.

In the long run, the organization may want to have about 1 percent of the professional staff trained at the black belt level and about 4 or 5 percent trained as green belts.

A typical on-site training program runs for one week, with the trainees taken away from their regular duties for essentially all of that week. By the end of that time, each person will have been assigned a training project to complete during the balance of the month. The trainer will be on call during that month to coach the trainees as necessary. The group meets again for one or two days to review the projects, straighten out any difficulties, and award green belts to successful participants.

Trainees pursuing the black belt will repeat the process, with another week of additional classroom training followed by a more substantial project that typically runs for another month. At the end of that second month, successful participants will be awarded the black belt.

Black belts who take a keen interest in Six Sigma may wish to pursue the master black belt at a training facility or through an online training company. Master black belts need more of a mathematical background or experience in statistical analysis as well as an interest in teaching others.

Many companies provide Six Sigma training, although few have specialized in healthcare issues. Most do industrial training, with an emphasis on factory performance. Many Six Sigma consulting companies will perform Six Sigma projects on a fee basis; some do both training and consulting. Relatively few have consulting experience in healthcare, although the number is growing.

This book includes a large number of healthcare cases, in part because healthcare training material is not available to any extent elsewhere. The 20-plus cases in this book provide sufficient case-study material for training green belts and black belts.

General Electric's Six Sigma Program

GE has embraced Six Sigma throughout its giant corporation, requiring all management candidates to be at least green belts. The company has an informative website at www.ge.com/sixsigma.

Most Six Sigma training companies and consulting companies have websites; any standard web search engine will identify them. Interested organizations may also contact the authors for training and consultation with specialization in healthcare.

Error Prevention

Errors are prevented by having the right equipment, the right infrastructure, trained personnel, and work tasks that lend themselves to being done correctly.

Errors are also prevented by managing the flow of work through the organization so that individual units are not overwhelmed by surges in demand. Hospital workflow has been getting attention recently with regard to both improving resource utilization and improving patient satisfaction (Mango and Shapiro 2001). Our attention is focused on understanding workflow principles to reduce the opportunity for error, which complements both resource utilization and patient satisfaction.

POKA-YOKE

Poka-yoke (Shingo 1981), pronounced po' kah yo' kay, is the Japanese term for mistake-proofing. The Japanese name has caught on because it has a better ring to it than the traditional American terms (fool-proofing, idiot-proofing, and the like), all of which are pejorative. Poka-yoke, being inscrutable, carries no negative connotation.

Poka-yoke is the fruit of a hundred years' study of the design of jobs and tasks. The results are these few guidelines, which are the essence of poka-yoke:

1. Make it easier for the person to do the right thing than the wrong thing.
2. Make mistakes obvious to the person immediately.
3. Allow the person to take corrective action on the spot.

Poka-yoke can also be seen as a systematic reduction of worker stress. Thinking that reduction of worker stress will mean a reduction in the worker's error rate is not rash. Getting this to work is not trivial, although the guidelines are quite simple. Take, for example, childproof caps for pill bottles. Their purpose is noble and fits exactly with the concepts of poka-yoke: They make it easier for the person in question (the child) to do the right thing (stay out of the pill bottle) than the wrong thing (get into the pill bottle). The difficulty arises in finding some cap design that keeps children out while still allowing adults to get to the pills. Because no single design for childproof caps exists, the adult wishing to open a new bottle must first figure out how this particular cap is supposed to work. Some are baffling; others require the adult to push down on the cap while turning it, which invites spilling the pills onto the floor or into the sink. The upshot may be that the bottle, once opened, is left open, which defeats the whole childproofing purpose.

Childproof caps are designed by very clever people working with unlimited budgets. Even so, the state of the art is wanting. This is offered as a cautionary tale and demonstrates that poka-yoke is not yet a settled practice of instant solutions.

Using terms like "design of work tasks" conveys the notion that, once a task is suitably designed, the matter is settled. This rarely happens, because things continue to change. Although most changes are incremental and the employee can make simple accommodations, measuring performance over time is a good practice so that any negative features that creep in are detected and dealt with in a timely manner, which is to say, before they get to be serious.

Poka-Yoke

Poka-yoke translates to "prevention of error by inadvertent action."

The older Japanese term was *baka-yoke*, which translates to "prevention of foolish action."

VERBAL ORDERS

Much of medical practice relies on verbal orders, commonly from doctor to nurse. Sometimes, the doctor misspeaks; sometimes, the nurse misunderstands.

If immediate feedback is given, the second poka-yoke guideline takes effect because the error is then obvious to the order giver. If the surgeon says "scalpel" and the nurse hands over forceps, immediate, tangible feedback is given. The error gets corrected right away, and no harm is done other than a slight delay. Note that the same corrective mechanism works even if the surgeon *thinks* "scalpel" but misspeaks and says "forceps." Whichever party makes the goof, the system makes the error obvious and easy to correct on the spot. Good poka-yoke.

Now, if the situation is different and does not provide immediate feedback, poka-yoke is not being followed and trouble may lurk. Suppose the physician says "Drug A" and the nurse hears "Drug B." Or, the physician thinks "Drug A" but says "Drug B." No feedback results, and the error could go undetected for too long a time.

Many organizations outside of healthcare run on verbal orders. The navies of the world have a way of generating feedback in exactly this situation. The captain gives an order to the lieutenant, who immediately repeats it, providing the necessary feedback to make poka-yoke work. Indeed, the navy order is repeated over and over again as the order passes down the chain of command. Then the response comes back up the chain of command, repeated several times. This is done even if the officers are standing side by side.

Curiously, neither the US Army nor the US Air Force follows this practice. Should they?

TOPICS IN ERROR PREVENTION IN HEALTHCARE

Here we will consider the poka-yoke principles as they apply to topics germane to healthcare organizations.

Personalization

Walmart has great big stores. Sam Walton, the founder of Walmart, decided that shoppers were finding his stores too impersonal. Because shoppers have other choices, Walton wanted to encourage shoppers to use his stores rather than those of others, so he worked to take the impersonal edge off. He hired people to stand at the door and greet shoppers as they came in, hand them shopping carts, offer a big smile (the Japanese version is to have employees stand at the door and bow deeply as customers come into the store; Americans smile better than we bow), and generally be personable. The point was to make the shopper feel welcome, to personalize an impersonal experience, and to take a little stress out of the situation.

Poka-Yoke Guidelines

Take the following steps to eliminate error:

1. Make doing the task right easier than doing it wrong.
2. Make errors immediately obvious.
3. Make the correction of errors on the spot possible.

Many healthcare organizations appear to be going the other way. Common practice today seems to be to have the patient interact with a clipboard: sign in here, mark the time, take a seat. This is now observed in general practices, in expensive specialists' offices, and in units within hospitals. This first interaction with the patient, who is already under some degree of stress, conveys the notion that the patient is not worth any personal attention. If the patient has questions great or small (Did I park in the right lot?), they are not important enough to merit attention. The patient is told to take a seat and wait.

Would Sam Walton run a medical service this way? Because the labor cost savings is obviously trivial, the patient gets the immediate impression that the organization thinks it is not getting a satisfactory amount of insurance money and is cutting corners by firing the receptionist. If you are the patient, you think the doctor is mad at you even before you get in the door. You, the patient, may begin to think, If the organization is cutting corners in the reception area, where else are corners being cut?

Instead of taking stress out of the situation the way Walmart does, these healthcare organizations are increasing the stress on the patient. This does not decrease the likelihood of error: The likelihood of error surely is higher. Not poka-yoke.

Buildings

Hospitals are trying to find ways for their big buildings to interact with patients and visitors. Some are using language-free signs, a good idea for our diverse society. Once understood, symbols are easy to recognize and interpret, even if the symbols are complex or abstract; the difficulty is figuring out what they mean the first time. Airlines have the same issue, and they deal with it by providing pamphlets in several languages to explain what the symbols mean.

Effective signage follows the first poka-yoke guideline by making it easier to get to the target destination on the first try. If taking the second poka-yoke guideline to heart, signs should also be placed where those who have wandered off the path will see them and discover immediately that they missed a turn. Following the third poka-yoke guideline allows the wanderer to correct the navigation error and get back on track.

Training for the Exceptional Event

Ralph Waldo Emerson (1860) wrote, "A great part of courage is the courage of having done the thing before." One hopes that healthcare workers do not need to call upon their courage very often, but the thought does extend to dealing with exceptional events. If the worker has dealt with the same event before, he or she is more likely to do the right thing. Being prepared makes doing the right thing easier, which very much complies with poka-yoke.

Airline pilots train for exceptional events with the use of flight simulators, which can create all manner of exceptional situations for the pilot to handle. The simulators are multimillion-dollar investments, the training time is extensive and recurring, and simulator staff salary is expensive. Those of us who fly from time to time are happy to know that the pilots and the airlines are, in their own interest, making it easier for the pilot to do the right thing rather than the wrong thing should one such exceptional event happen in real life.

Anesthesiologists are now training with computerized mannequins (Gaba, Fish, and Howard 1994) so that they will have "done it before" and thus be prepared when some low-occurrence event presents itself in real life. Other medical specialties are also researching the applications of computerized mannequins. Presently such training is conducted for one specialist at a time, although the extension of training to the whole surgery team or to other teams of caregivers would seem to be straightforward and beneficial.

Nurses and emergency medical personnel use mannequins for cardiopulmonary resuscitation training, water rescue drills, and the like. Mannequins that can generate a range of cardiac patterns on the electrocardiography monitor are used for advanced cardiac life-support training. This is all quite positive, and further extension of this training technology would be even better.

Many healthcare organizations carry out disaster drills, which heretofore were commonly designed to consider some industrial disaster appropriate for the area. Currently, disaster drills for terrorist actions are a clear and present need. Companies with offices in the World Trade Center who had taken their fire drills seriously beforehand are now believed to have fared better in the tragedy on September 11, 2001, than those who had not; clearly, the words of Emerson and the concepts of poka-yoke ring true in this example. Large-scale drills are good both as a means to gain some practice and as a means to develop workflow data for management to consider.

Repetition

When it comes to error frequency, people follow a bathtub curve. We make mistakes during the early stages as we acquire the skills to perform any task. A long flat period follows when mistakes almost never happen. Later, the error rate rises again as people develop bad habits. The flat period can be extended by periodic retraining. For example, airline pilots do periodic simulator retraining even though they fly the same plane every day. Some healthcare certifications require periodic demonstration that the skills are still there; sometimes the same training mannequins are used again. This is good counter–bathtub curve practice. Consideration should be given to extending this to other skills, both those that are used infrequently and those that are used frequently. Again, another demonstration of poka-yoke.

Healthcare practitioners, as a rule, perform many tasks—even complicated ones—from memory rather than by following a checklist. Airline pilots follow a checklist every time they take the plane off the ground, even if they take off and land six times a day. Which of these professionals is less likely to skip a step or do things out of sequence? Which is better protected from the bathtub curve? Which practice is in adherence of poka-yoke?

Keying and Interlocks

We use "keying" in the sense of a key used to solve a puzzle. Color, size, shape, weight, and feel are keys that contribute to a person selecting the right object, such as a pill or instrument, and recognizing quickly if he or she has made the wrong selection. Keying shows good poka-yoke.

Interlocks take the decision out of the person's hands and may or may not be a good idea. The earlier example of childproof caps describes an interlock. Five-drawer file cabinets are another type of interlock. They are commonly designed so that only one drawer can be open at a time; this is done for the good reason that the cabinet is apt to fall over on the person pulling on the drawers if the top two drawers are open at the same time. Airlocks between public rooms and controlled-atmosphere rooms are other interlocks. Interlocks such as these that deal with only one function are generally good ideas.

The question becomes much more difficult if multiple functions are involved. For example, fire hydrants have large bolt heads that are to be turned to permit the water to flow, and the bolt heads have five sides rather than the customary six. This has been done so that a standard wrench will not fit and only the five-sided wrench carried by firemen on the truck will. This is another example of an interlock, and in this case it is used to prevent children from playing with the fire hydrant. But what happens if a legitimate need for water arises and no fire truck is on hand? A day may come when more fires occur than trucks are available to fight them. In that event, how will the supply of water be accessed?

Kitting

Preparing burn kits, gallbladder kits, appendectomy kits, and others is poka-yoke because it makes it easy to have the right set of supplies on hand when a specific treatment is to be performed. The kitting can be completed at a time of less stress or even by the suppliers. If the kitting is done in-house, providing a key such as a yellow tag when the kit is incomplete is important. Shelf life needs to be evident. Kitting can be extended to all kinds of services, even to the preparation of insurance forms.

Kits are inventory. Some judgment is required when deciding which kits to make up and which ones are not necessary. If the organization sees one case of lion fever every 20 years, a lion fever kit would not seem to be a good use of working capital.

Computer Displays

Computer displays can generate information overload. The trend—and it is a good one—is to simplify computer displays, to use more diagrammatic presentations, to prioritize alarms, and to make the information understandable to the nonspecialist.

Specialists who understand the complex displays will generally say that the displays are just fine the way they are. The complex displays allow the specialists to apply their mastery and preserve the special knowledge they have acquired. The experts do not see a need for any help, and they do not want any help.

In fields other than healthcare, giving the experts help, even if they do not want it, is found to reduce error rates. You may have seen the ground control room NASA uses at the Johnson Space Center for space shuttle launches and now for Space Station Freedom. It is a big room with lots of desks, computer displays, and telephones, and it is filled with experts doing important, life-critical tasks. NASA has been operating such rooms for more than 50 years and has learned something about computer–expert interfaces. As computers have become more powerful over the years, NASA has upgraded the computer displays, adding more information but also reorganizing and reprioritizing the information so that less-expert humans can understand what is going on. Because of this, NASA has found that the error rate—of errors made by experts—has gone down and turnover has gone up. These positions, which now require less expertise, are less attractive to the engineering staff. The important thing, though, is that the error rate has gone down.

Perhaps this is the case in the healthcare field, too: Even though experts do not want the help, maybe they could use a little anyway, for the good of the cause. Computer displays should make doing the right thing easier than doing the wrong thing by organizing the pertinent information and guiding the person to do the right thing. They should make it obvious, immediately, when the wrong thing has been done. Computer displays should allow a person a second chance by allowing him or her to recover from an error before irreversible action is taken. All of these ideas are not only common sense, they are poka-yoke.

Fatigue

Tired people make mistakes. Physical and mental conditioning can help, but the body eventually runs out of gas. In emergencies, fatigue is unavoidable. In everyday operations, on the other hand, fatigue should be avoided by suitable policies. Requiring nurses to work double shifts is inviting mistakes; having staff on call for extended periods is inviting mistakes. Airline pilots may work long flights, but once they are on the ground, they are required by law to stay on the ground until they have had a full eight hours at their hotel.

Essential Equipment

Essential equipment should have sufficient backups on hot standby or cold standby, with the backup equipment checked out and ready to go in the same manner as the primary equipment. The reliability of the combined systems should be at least 99.999,999 percent.

The equipment should display its status and let the user know what is going on inside. Modern computerized devices act more and more like black boxes, keeping their doings quite secret. Good design shows a running report or display of what the device is doing at every moment so that the user will know the machine is working and doing things that seem to be reasonable.

System Reliability

High system reliability can be achieved by providing two or three systems in parallel or as backups. Three systems with 99.9, 99.9, and 99.0 percent reliability rates combine to attain "eight-nines reliability"; just add the nines of the individual systems. This works as long as they have no common modes of failure. A system with eight-nines reliability is expected to be out of service less than one second per year.

Status of Work

The status of all work needs to be evident so that, if some mistake is made, that mistake is evident. For example, putting an X-ray into the viewer in a reversed position is an easy mistake to make. No keying can prevent this error, and the occurrence of this error is not obvious to the technician. This goes against the poka-yoke guidelines. Why are X-ray films not stamped "FRONT" and "BACK" in large letters, or perhaps "RECTO" and "VERSO"? How about a color key?

Patient Location

A particular status issue is the location of each patient. Is the patient in bed? Did the patient get out of bed? The second poka-yoke guideline says that mistakes should be evident so that they can be corrected. If the patient got out of bed on his or her own, contrary to instructions, how is the care staff going to know? If the patient decides to leave the care unit on his or her own, how is the care staff going to know? Is every baby in the nursery where it is supposed to be?

Patient Identification

Patient identification bracelets are helpful, but they are not quite perfect. Biometric devices such as retina and face scanners may provide more direct identification in the near future. These scanners require no contact with the person, which would be an advantage over fingerprint scanners, as it reduces the potential spread of germs. Until some such absolute identification system is practicable, satisfying the poka-yoke guideline to recognize errors immediately will be difficult if the error is in identification. Until such biometric devices are available, what special steps should be taken to reconfirm patient identification before any irreversible action?

Pause

Ideally, the worker should be able to pause at any time to take stock for a few moments. Did I do everything? Does this look right? Feel right? Sound right? Is everything on hand for the next step? This ideal may seem like too much to ask, but it is generally possible to design the work plan to build in a pause before each irreversible step.

Allowing for a pause implies no synchronous operations. If Worker A has to keep up with Worker B or Machine C, then Worker A does not have a meaningful opportunity to inject a pause. Because of this, synchronous operations should be avoided. However, this does not exclude parallel operations. Keep in mind that each parallel operation should have points that allow for a pause so that other operations can catch up.

Recovery

It would be great if a person could identify an error and recover from it with no harm or risk to the patient or any other damage done. This is possible if the number of irreversible steps is few and things are checked carefully before each of those irreversible steps. Again, the concepts of poka-yoke should always be kept in mind.

Stopping the Line

It took more than 50 years, but manufacturers eventually came to understand that every worker, even the one who seems least important, needs to be able to stop the assembly line if something is amiss; it is better to stop the line occasionally for a false alarm than to continue with errors. Because of this belief, stop buttons are now placed all over factories. Claxons sound, and much attention is rendered. Decisions are made, corrections are made if necessary, and then the line starts up again.

Healthcare does not often run on an assembly line, but the message is the same. Consideration should be given to empowering *all* employees to raise questions, point out unusual conditions, and get respectful attention. In high-stress situations, interjections are not automatically welcomed, which is why it took so long to get to this level of understanding even in the "low-stress" factory. This ideal working environment takes time and effort to achieve. It is a good idea, though, and it is poka-yoke, because even the most insignificant-seeming worker is acting on a perceived error in an effort to prevent the error from continuing to happen.

Accounting

Accounting errors are just as aggravating as treatment errors. A particular feature of accounting errors is that they are commonly made by people who do not know they are making an error and consequently cannot remedy the error on the spot. In many cases, the data input to the accounting program is not done by the person who has performed the work but rather by someone else working with secondhand or thirdhand information.

Newer systems that use barcode readers in the patient care unit, in the laboratory, in the pharmacy, and in other places avoid this particular weakness of traditional accounting systems. However, the newer systems do not usually reach poka-yoke goals because no feedback is given to the person operating the barcode reader. A beep may well sound to indicate that the barcode was digested, but there is rarely a report back to that person to show what the effect on the accounting statement turned out to be. This invites the possibility of doubled entries that are not likely to be spotted until the patient does the spotting.

Good poka-yoke practice is to use live data entry by the worker and to feed the accounting result back immediately to the person who is doing the work. That way, the person who actually knows something about the situation can look to see if the accounting entry is right and, if it is not, recognize the error on the spot so that some corrective action can be taken while the event is still fresh in the mind.

Case Administration

Each patient's case involves treatment coding, releases, and other administrative actions, nearly all of which are done by people who are not standing next to the patient. This means that errors can be made that are not immediately obvious; thus, application of the poka-yoke guidelines is difficult.

Untimely administrative actions are also errors because they may delay the treatment or discharge of a patient. Creating an administrative system that encourages timely administrative actions is particularly difficult, in healthcare or in any other kind of organization. Management is left with the responsibility for creating an administrative system with a sufficient number of checks built in but without the benefit of feedback that occurs naturally in the caregiving parts of the organization. The combined system should be built on the poka-yoke guidelines: Right decisions should be easier to make than wrong ones, errors should be immediately obvious, and correction should be possible on the spot. Timeliness should also be considered. How can the system be designed so that decisions are made as soon as they are ripe rather than some time later? Are the right incentives in place? Is the right information flow happening? Do the decision makers and the decision bases come together at the right time? Are there policy impediments? Do the decision makers even know when the decision is ripe? If they make the wrong decision, how and when do they find out about it? How do they correct errors on the spot?

Buildings and Infrastructure

Fire zones, quarantine zones, isolation zones, and the like all need to be tested. Personnel access to restricted zones needs to be challenged by such means as having tame outsiders try to penetrate the zones. Such innocent intruders are a better test of a system than any number of paper studies.

Electric backup systems must be ready to go. Diesel generators need to be started periodically and run under load. The reliability of the combined system should not be less than 99.999,999 percent.

Communications systems these days include landline telephones, wireless radios, and computer networks. Although the combined reliability of these systems can be expected to be quite high (often better than 99.999,999 percent), communications systems are prone to hidden common modes of failure. Building telephone connections to two separate central offices is good practice, but make sure the two connections are not hung on the same poles or run through the same trenches. Wireless telephone calls might be routed through the same central office as the landline phones, the data network might run through the same central office or use the same poles or trenches, and even radio traffic might be going through the same central offices; the only way to find out is to have the several communications contractors walk their lines and report back to you.

Data networks are subject to attack by pranksters and villains. This is a matter for data network specialists, and it needs to be taken seriously. Having tame outsiders "attack" the data network can be most illuminating. Because the attack techniques seem to be evolving continually, this is an abiding concern that will be with us until somebody figures out how to make a secure data network. The same applies for water supplies, drains, special gases, and other systems important to patient care. The status of the essential building services should be displayed at all times, not only for the plant engineer but for senior management as well.

Poka-yoke comes into play in the design and operation of these infrastructure systems. First, the fundamental design needs to be free from hidden error, and the operating panels and control stations need to be designed so that doing the right thing is always easier than doing the wrong thing. Second, the poka-yoke guidelines say that errors—or, in this case, off-normal conditions—need to be evident so they can be redressed. Third, the design of the systems needs to be such that the operator can easily recover from any error.

Medication

Medication errors are thought to be among the most common serious errors in healthcare and include errors made during the writing of the prescription, dispensing by the pharmacy, handling by staff, and handling by the patient in self-medicating circumstances (Joint Commission 2016a).

The first poka-yoke guideline obviously applies to getting the right prescription rather than the wrong one. The second and third poka-yoke guidelines apply not only to the physician but also to everybody else in the chain. How can the pharmacist spot a possible error? How can the staff nurse spot an error at the patient's bedside? How can the patient, sent home with a list of medications, spot an error? If the patient does something wrong at home, how does that patient recognize the error and know what remedial action to take?

Computerized physician orders, computerized crosschecking by the pharmacist, and barcode tracking of medication and patient all go in the right direction, but they focus only on the first guideline and do not do much in the way of making evident those few errors that creep through the checks, and they do nothing to facilitate recovery actions. For the discharged patient self-medicating at home, the situation is less structured, and control is lacking. Still, thoughtful application of poka-yoke may provide some help. Predischarge training of the patient and the at-home family care provider can help. Postdischarge retraining by visiting nurses can also help.

This pre- and postdischarge training should cover all three of the poka-yoke guidelines, addressing

1. how to organize the medication and schedule to make taking the right medicine at the right time easier than taking the wrong medicine or taking it at the wrong time,
2. how to recognize an error on the spot, and
3. what to do when an error is made.

Covering the first of these guidelines when designing training plans is natural. However, covering the second and third will take some conscious thought because it may be construed as detracting from the primary message, which is, "Do this the way I am telling you to do it." Still, people make mistakes, and the second and third guidelines need to be part of the patient training package.

The Tell-Tale

Some actions have no obvious effect, so the second poka-yoke guideline cannot be applied. In these cases, the person cannot immediately tell if the action was done correctly or if it was even done at all. In addition, it is not obvious how any supervisor can verify that the action was taken in such situations. For instance, certain patients are supposed to be moved about in their wheelchairs every two hours to prevent pressure ulcers; however, it is hard to know whether this action has taken place every time.

Adding a tell-tale might help. A tell-tale is any feature that tells the tale, such as a little flag on the wheelchair, red on one side and yellow on the other, that is reversed each time the patient's position is adjusted. Before-and-after photographs would work, too, and would create a permanent record. Clipboard check-off goes in the same direction, although this method tends to receive less diligent attention. Other situations that are difficult to observe also pose challenges. Did Mrs. Jones take her after-dinner pills, or did she slip them in among the food remnants on the tray?

Employee Security

The rate of assaults on healthcare workers is five times as high as that on workers in general, and injuries and deaths do occur (Gribbin 2002; OSHA 2013). An injury to an employee is of the same gravity as injury to a patient, and prevention steps need to be taken.

Poka-yoke can perhaps be of some assistance in the design of policies to increase the likelihood of making the right decision when identifying threats posed by patients and others and taking preventive measures such as restraints and physical barriers when the risk is nonnegligible.

Many questions must be considered. How can the person who poses a threat of assault be identified? Must there be a prior record? Physical indicators? Warnings received? How is an error in identification recognized as quickly as possible? Have menacing actions or threats been made? How can an error in identification be recovered from, before damage is done? Are escape routes or guards nearby?

This is a troubling subject, and the needs of organizations vary widely. Perhaps the poka-yoke discipline can be of some assistance, although poka-yoke targets inadvertent error, not malicious error.

Detecting and Visualizing Problems

*Detecting abnormal conditions before they become problems
is better than waiting for untoward events to happen.*

*Problem detection requires that a baseline be established and quantified,
that ongoing data be gathered and tracked, and that warning levels be
established so that abnormal data can be flagged and studied in detail.*

*Management may become aware of abnormal conditions through
anecdotal reports. Taking action to correct such conditions
usually works better if quantitative information is in hand.*

WHAT TO DO WITH DATA BEFORE DOING ANYTHING WITH DATA

Modern spreadsheets make visualization easy—so easy that that's the place to start with every project. To make evidence-based decisions, one must visualize the evidence.

Consider a small primary care practice with seven doctors, all of whom see the same mix of patients. The exhibits that follow are based on all the doctors seeing 50 patients each over the same period of time. Experimenting with various ways of displaying the data graphically helps highlight patterns and convey information. Modern spreadsheets display an instant chart as the cursor floats over the wide selection of chart possibilities, helping the eye identify a format quickly to organize the data in the best way.

One chart style that seems to be interesting is a histogram (see exhibit 4.1) of all patients seen by all doctors—that is, 7 doctors times 50 patients each, making 350 patients total.

Exhibit 4.1: Histogram of Consultation Times for Seven Doctors

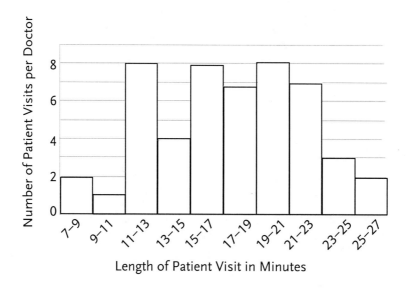

This histogram looks vaguely like a normal distribution, which seems reasonable. On the left end of the horizontal axis, the first "bin" ranges not from zero to something but from seven to nine. While a few patient visits last from seven to nine minutes, no visit lasts less than seven. Perhaps that means the doctors are occupied with setup and preparation for five or six minutes in every case. It might be worth asking if some of that preparation work could be done by a nurse or clerk. If so, doctors might be able to devote more time to each patient and perhaps see more patients in total.

There are only a few patients in the first two bins on the left. If the first six minutes are for preparation, then these patients were only seen for a couple of minutes. Very likely they were sent back out the door, and it seems equally likely that these patients could have been screened beforehand and not placed in the doctor's queue.

On the right side of the chart, we find just a few patients requiring more than 23 minutes. For scheduling purposes, perhaps these few would be ignored, after further examination of the particulars of those cases.

Exhibit 4.1, formatted as a histogram, lumps all patients into one pile. There may be something more to observe in a chart that brings out the differences among the seven doctors. Consider a box-and-whiskers chart such as exhibit 4.2.

Exhibit 4.2: Box Chart of Consultation Times for Seven Doctors

The box covers half the data for each doctor, the whiskers are the vertical lines stretching from the high to the low values, and any tiny circles would indicate data that are exceptions, well away from the rest. A horizontal line through the box marks the mean.

The essence of Six Sigma is to find and eliminate variability that is not essential, to preclude the masking of important information.

The sizes of the boxes look about the same for all seven doctors, so box size may represent the variability intrinsic to the mix of patients. The low whisker is pretty close to 10 minutes for five of the doctors, but the seventh doctor's low whisker is higher, and the third doctor's low whisker is higher still. All doctors are seeing the same mix of patients, so maybe doctors three and seven take more time getting started with a new patient. Doctor seven recovers so that the average completion time is pretty good and competitive with the others. However, doctor three's whole figure is higher on the page, meaning that for this provider, the slower start leads to longer completion times.

It is to be noted that, in this box-and-whisker chart, nothing much happens in less than 10 minutes, which is another way of observing that doctors may be spending quite a bit of time on preparation that could be delegated to a nurse, clerk, or physician's assistant.

Exhibit 4.2 reveals three exceptions, two of which are favorable and one that is unfavorable. Doctors one and six appear to get the work done more expeditiously, while doctor three lags. Exceptions are rich in information, so it is useful to investigate each one and determine its cause.

These doctors see patients consecutively, and it is to be expected that consultation times would average out. To see if that makes much difference, the total completion times for two consecutive patients have been calculated (by adding rows one and two, three and four, etc.) and new charts created. We'll start with a new box-and-whisker chart, shown in exhibit 4.3.

Exhibit 4.3: Box Chart of Consecutive Consultations

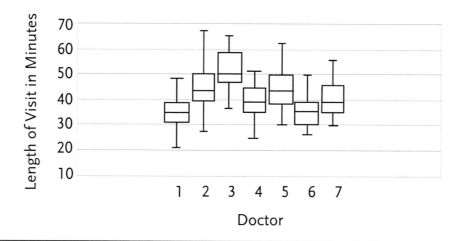

Here, the data are a little closer together, vertically, but not much. Doctor three still catches the eye.

Perhaps a look at all the consultation times of all the doctors together might reveal something. Exhibit 4.4 shows a composite histogram of the time for two consecutive patients, using the same data as before.

This histogram shows that only a few consecutive cases require more than 41 minutes. Knowing this helps plan for periods of peak demand.

Exhibit 4.4: Histogram of Consecutive Consultations

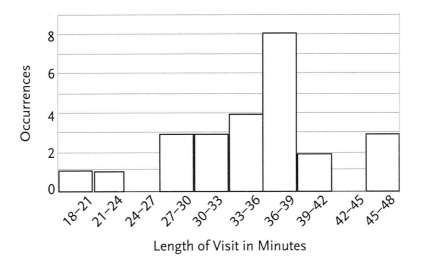

GO LOOK

Waiting rooms are filled with information. Sitting in one to see what goes on can reveal a lot. Do people come early or late to appointments? Do any of them leave? Do people seem to know what to do and where to find things? Are clerks visible and providing help? Are there employees wandering through?

Follow a few patients all the way through the system. How are they treated at each point? How are they getting information? Any language problems? Any missed steps? Any misunderstandings?

SIX SIGMA MEASURES

For ongoing operations, measure the overall system error rate and the variability of the error rate. Because most organizations provide several treatments or services, keeping track of error rates and variability for each one makes sense. We will also most often be interested in the error rate, and its variability, for each work unit involved in each service. As a measure of variability, we will track the standard deviation of each item of interest.

We will commonly keep track of the time duration involved in each step and its variability. There is no Six Sigma goal for variability, but tracking variability is important because the variability plays into the ongoing analysis of each process.

Six Sigma organizations seek to perform at an error rate of 3.4 errors per million opportunities. How many opportunities for error does a healthcare service organization encounter? For present purposes, assume that a professional employee does something five to ten times an hour, and that each attempt at a process might go wrong or be delayed. For every 100 professional employees, that equates to one to two million opportunities for error in a year. Nonprofessionals, being more task-oriented, would likely have 15 to 30 opportunities for error per hour. Every 100 non-professionals, then, would have three to six million opportunities for error per year.

That said, an organization of 500 people, with 150 professionals and 350 non-professionals, would have about one to two million opportunities for error per month. If this organization were applying Six Sigma successfully, the number of errors for the whole organization would be fewer than ten per month. Even a very good organization operating in the best known mode will still have errors cropping up, because having perfection in service is not possible by any known means. However, those rare errors will be found and corrected promptly in an ongoing, managed way.

HOW ARE WE DOING?

Studies show that American industry is presently running at about four sigma and that service organizations are running at one to two sigma (Breyfogle, Cupello, and Meadows 2000). How big is a sigma? What does "four sigma" or "one to two sigma" performance mean?

Here's an example. In 2013, the government reports that the Centers for Medicare & Medicaid Services paid out money with a 10 percent error rate, equivalent to some $50 billion paid out in error (Healthcare Finance Staff 2013). That's a success rate of 1.3 sigma for this service operation. One might hope for better.

The symbol σ, or sigma, represents the standard deviation of a distribution of possible occurrences. The most familiar distribution is the normal distribution, which is that familiar bell-shaped curve. The normal curve is plotted against the number of standard deviations; the curve is symmetric in relation to its average value. The normal curve is one of those curves that

American Experience

- Industry: Four sigma
- Services: One to two sigma

Source: Breyfogle, Cupello, and Meadows (2000).

Exhibit 4.5: Normal Distribution with Tail

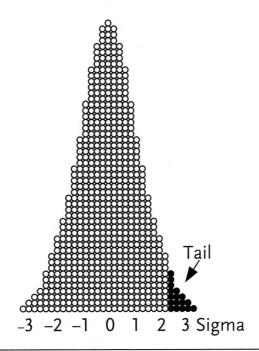

never quite gets to zero: No matter how far along the sigma-axis one goes, a little more tail continues to the right, and the same is true for the left side of the curve, which is for the negative values of sigma (see exhibit 4.5, which is probably familiar). Sometimes both tails are of interest, and sometimes only one side or the other is.

The present matter of interest is how much of a tail corresponds to a particular sigma value. The tail is the area under the normal curve to the right of the sigma value. To show some specific numbers, here are the tails for a selection of sigma values:

	Tail	
Sigma Value	Items per Thousand	Items per Million
1	159	158,665
2	23	22,750
3	1	1,350
4		32
4.5		3.4

A system running at the one-sigma level experiences 159 errors per 1,000 opportunities, a system running at the two-sigma level experiences 23 errors per 1,000 opportunities, and a system running at the three-sigma level experiences about 1 error per 1,000 opportunities.

For higher sigma values, it is more convenient to present the number of errors per million opportunities. A system running at the three-sigma level is experiencing 1,350 errors per million, a system running at the four-sigma level experiences 32 errors per million, and a system running at the 4.5-sigma level experiences 3.4 errors per million.

Six Sigma organizations want to be so sure that the goal of 3.4 errors per million is met that, rather than setting 4.5 sigma as the goal, the bar is set at a full six sigma; this allows 1.5 sigma for process variation. Process variation may arise from normal turnover in work crews, the time needed to gain familiarity with new equipment, the addition of new services, and the like. Making some allowances for such common process variations is considered more prudent than having to explain shortfalls later on.

Returning to our hypothetical healthcare organization with 500 employees, the number of opportunities for error is one to two million per month, so the number of errors for the organization per month would be as follows:

Sigma	Organization Errors per Month	
	Low	High
1	158,000	317,000
2	22,750	45,500
3	1,350	2,700
4	32	63
4.5	3.4	6.8

If service organizations are running between one and two sigma these days, then the 500-person organization would be experiencing perhaps 100,000 errors per month. That's a lot—it's about 200 errors per person per month, or about one error per person every hour.

Suppose our organization is better than average, running at 2.5 sigma, which would be about 10,000 errors per month, which can also be stated as 20 errors per person per month or about one error per person per day. On the other hand, if our organization were achieving 4.5 sigma, the entire organization would be making about five errors per month, which would be 0.01 errors per person per month, or one error per person every eight years or so.

The improvement for our hypothetical organization would be from several thousand errors per month to fewer than ten per month. The improvement would be reflected directly in improved service to patients and in a direct reduction in the cost, capacity, and management effort presently applied to correcting errors and dealing with the consequences of errors.

Even if as few as one or two errors per person per day occur, it is not difficult to imagine that 10 percent of the total effort goes into correcting mistakes. If the organization is presently putting 10 percent of its resources into error and the consequences of error, the organization stands to recover nearly all of that misapplication of its resources, and that savings goes directly to the bottom line.

An error is any departure from specification. For example, the specification may be that a service department perform on a particular time schedule, within a stated time window. Failure to perform within this time window counts as an error. Or, suppose certain laboratory reports are part of a healthcare service and that the system is set up to tolerate report turnaround with an average of four hours and a range from three to five hours. Timely delivery of these reports is important to the completion of the patient's care; anything earlier causes confusion, and anything later causes delays.

On the left-hand side of exhibit 4.6, the laboratory is meeting the requirement and honoring the established service window in time. This meets the Crosby definition of quality because the specification is met.

Exhibit 4.6: Inconsistent and Consistent Performance

Arrival Times

Arrival Times

On the right-hand side of exhibit 4.6, the laboratory is doing a little more by delivering the reports on a consistent basis very near the nominal average delivery time. This meets the Crosby definition and does something more: It fulfills the requirements with great consistency. Meeting specifications with consistency is an embellishment on the Crosby quality requirement that was expanded by Taguchi (1978) and is a good goal to keep in mind.

If one had the choice, one would certainly choose to appear on the right-hand side of the exhibit, the side that represents consistent performance. With that level of performance, the receiving department will have more confidence that the next report will arrive within the specified time window.

SIX SIGMA OPERATIONS ANALYSIS

System Yield and Performance Time

Multistep Performance

The overall yield is the product of the yields of each of the steps.

The overall performance time is the sum of the performance times of each of the steps.

The yield is the ratio of desired outcomes to total outcomes.

The *system yield* is the ratio of the number of everything-right-the-first-time patients to the total number of patients treated. The system yield is also the product of the yields of each step in the overall process.

The *system performance time* is the time needed to complete the treatment and discharge the patient. The system performance time is also the sum of the treatment times of each step in the overall process plus any waiting time.

The system yield has an average value and a standard deviation; so does the system performance time. Most healthcare organizations provide more than one service, so there would be a yield and a performance time for each service.

Example One

Suppose the system yield is 99.9 percent and the system performance time is 50 hours. That means the next patient could expect to move through the system in about 50 hours. Out of the next 1,000 patients, *one* can expect to require corrective action to overcome some error made inside the system. The number of patients in the system getting corrective action would be a tiny fraction of the whole patient population. This is good because resources devoted to that corrective action are resources that are not available for taking care of the next patient.

Example Two

Suppose now that the overall system yield is found to be 80 percent, with a standard deviation of 3 percent, and suppose that the overall system performance time is found to be 100 hours, with a standard deviation of 5 hours.

Any single patient can expect to be through the system in about 100 hours. Only one patient out of 1,000 will expect to take longer than 115 hours (the arithmetic will be developed in the following sections), and a few out of a million will take longer than 130 hours. These are patients who require no corrective action during the overall process; they are simply held up someplace along the line for more time than the average.

Because the yield is only 80 percent, a 20 percent chance exists that any one patient will be held up for additional work and that, out of several groups of patients, some groups may see as many as 29 percent of the group held up for additional work. In extremely rare cases, a group may see as many as 38 percent held up for additional work.

Clearly, having 20 percent of patients being given additional treatment means that a lot of the effort of the system is being given over to this additional corrective care. If this additional care involves the bottleneck of the system, the overall capacity of the system is reduced directly by this fraction. Therefore, management efforts to improve the yield at each process step will be rewarded by reducing the effort going into that additional care, and the capacity of the overall system will increase as less additional work flows through the bottleneck.

Example Three

The average treatment time is not known, and the yield is not known. Everybody seems happy, though, and nothing seems to get stuck in the middle. This is a good situation to leave alone. There are bound to be greater difficulties elsewhere.

Example Four

The average treatment time is not known, and the yield is not known. Complaints are coming in about work being redone, about work or patients piling up, and about unhappy employees. This scenario goes on the list for further examination. Something is wrong, and the management might as well find out what it is now rather than find out the hard way later. It is best to gather information and organize it so that informed decisions can be reached.

SIX SIGMA PROCESS ANALYSIS

Six Sigma provides an organized way of gathering and organizing information about ongoing processes by proceeding step by step:

1. Select key or troublesome processes.
2. Quantify present performance to have a baseline.

3. Evaluate candidate changes to improve the process.
4. Execute process improvements on a trial basis.
5. Extend successful trials to the organization.
6. Monitor the new process over the long term.
7. Select the next candidates for improvement.

There will always be another candidate process worthy of consideration because technology changes, the services that are offered change, personnel change, and outside factors, such as new regulations, come into play. Therefore, Six Sigma becomes an abiding feature of organizations that take up Six Sigma and find Six Sigma to be effective.

Six Sigma performance begins by gathering and organizing information. On the basis of this information, changes are considered and given a trial run in controlled circumstances. If these trials are successful, the change can be implemented widely. The ongoing monitoring that follows ensures that no deterioration goes undetected over time. In addition, the ongoing monitoring may bring to light some pattern of performance that is better than usual and that deserves closer attention as a potential benefit.

SIX SIGMA SYSTEM LIMITS

Each process's yield and duration have two characteristics: an average and a standard deviation. These two characteristics become the basis for quantitative analysis of the process.

The Six Sigma method establishes two *system limits* for each process: the upper system limit and the lower system limit. The system limits bracket the process outcomes from above and below. The space in between is called the *system limits band* or just the system band.

To make use of these limits, use tracking charts and plot data points on these charts against time. Draw a horizontal line to represent the average value, and draw the system limits six standard deviations away from the average value.

A process governed by a normal distribution will take on values more than 4.5 standard deviations away from the average only 3.4 times in a million. Because that is the numerical goal for Six Sigma, the logic for allowing 4.5 standard deviations of room for random fluctuations is easy to see. Six Sigma goes beyond this by allowing an additional 1.5 standard deviations for drift in the process average value. Adding 4.5 and 1.5 standard deviations gives 6 standard deviations. The system limits are drawn six standard deviations away from the average value; this is done separately for the process yield and the process duration. If the lower limit goes below zero, the lower limit is set to zero.

To see the reason for the additional 1.5 standard deviations of allowance, consider that it is prudent to allow some measure for the aging of equipment, variations in the weather, bringing new people into the work group, a change in suppliers, and every other ordinary reason that might come along. The system limits are pretty important, and changes in them may cause ripples throughout the organization; to be on the safe side, allow some leeway for these nonspecific influences. The size of the allowance is open for debate; American industry has found that an allowance of 1.5 standard deviations seems to be practical, and so 1.5 standard deviations has been adopted as part of the Six Sigma method.

To demonstrate this, exhibit 4.7 shows a typical normal distribution with the 3.4-per-million limits shown at plus and minus 4.5 standard deviations from the average value and the system limits marked at plus and minus 6 standard deviations.

Exhibit 4.7: Balanced Normal Distribution with System Limits

Balanced Normal Distribution

This normal distribution, as long as it stays where it is in the middle of the system band, will have fluctuations that reach the system limits much less often than 3.4 times per million because there is substantial white space between the 3.4-per-million limits and the system limits.

In the next chart (exhibit 4.8), the process, for some as-yet-unknown reason, has drifted somewhat to the right by about one standard deviation. The 3.4-per-million

Exhibit 4.8: Drifted Normal Distribution with System Limits

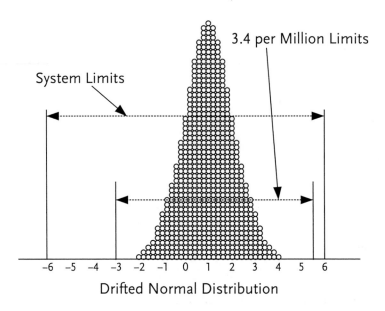

Drifted Normal Distribution

limits move with the distribution because these are simply characteristics of that distribution. The system limits, however, do not move; once they are set, they stay the same. In this case, because of the drift, the white space has largely been eaten up on the right-hand side. Although it may well be time to take action to rectify the situation, the built-in allowance provides a margin so that the system limits are not yet violated more than 3.4 times per million.

Why System Limits Are Important

The system limits for a process are a declaration to the overall system that says, "This is what I can do with great reliability. If you ask no more of me than this, I can perform to Six Sigma standards. If you ask more, I will likely fail to meet the Six Sigma standards. If you want tighter system limits, you will have to change the process."

The system limits are the interface between this process and the organization. Suppose the process in question is the X-ray department, and suppose that observations lead to the determination that the average time to provide an X-ray, once the patient is delivered to the X-ray department door, is 30 minutes with a standard deviation of 5 minutes. The upper system limit for X-ray completion time comes to $30 + (6 \times 5) = 60$ minutes. The patient care unit requesting the X-ray would need to plan sufficiently to allow for as much as 60 minutes for the X-ray so as not to be disappointed more than 3.4 times per million. Of the 60 minutes, 7.5 minutes are the white-space allowance for process drift over time.

The patient care unit would likely demand that the X-ray department pay attention and turn patients around a good deal more promptly than that, to which the X-ray department can say, "Yes, we would like to do better and we will consider ways to do better, but that is the process that exists today, and we do not know how to improve the process overnight, so you had better plan on 60 minutes until further notice."

Knowing the system limits provides a basis for rational management action at three places. Higher management can see the benefit of capital improvements or additional staffing in the X-ray department because it will have an observable benefit in treatment time. The X-ray department itself has a rational basis for putting forward capital and staffing requests. The patient care unit has a rational basis for planning its work on a reliable schedule.

Suppose the measure is not of X-ray completion time but rather of the incidence of lost X-rays, which result in the patient having to be returned to the X-ray department to be x-rayed again. If that happens frequently, the X-ray department must have the capacity to deal with the reshoots, the patient care unit must plan for the likelihood of reshoots, and the whole treatment process must make a suitable allowance. Having the system limits established provides a basis for deciding what to do in each of the affected units.

Process Tracking

Establishing the system limits once does not end the necessary interest in each process. Things change, so it is important to keep track of performance over time. The system limits are set so wide that they will not likely ever be violated in the normal course of events; indeed, that is the whole point. Therefore, it is generally helpful to establish an additional pair of limits, for tracking purposes, that are closer to where the data points are expected to fall.

The customary way of doing this is to set limits at plus and minus three standard deviations, which will be surpassed about one time in every 1,000. Crossing these lines does not violate anything; it simply puts the responsible people on notice that something unusual has happened. Maybe it is a random fluctuation, or maybe it is something going awry in the process. It is a data point worth some additional attention.

Limits set at plus and minus three standard deviations have the historical name of "process control limits," although nothing is being controlled in the usual sense of the word. (Nothing is "controlled" at a border passport-control office either, so using the word in this sense, to mean inspection or observation, is not unique.) When data points fall outside the process control limits, the mechanisms for problem solving, which were described earlier, can be applied. When data points fall outside the system limits, those mechanisms certainly should be applied.

A Pharmacy Order Example

Consider this hypothetical case. A hospital has a pharmacy, and the pharmacy fills medication orders from the patient care units. Experience shows that about one medication order in 1,000 is wrong; either the dosage level is wrong or the drug delivered is not the one intended. Management is concerned about this level of performance and decides to take action; an additional rechecking step is initiated to break the chain of events. Then management decides that additional information should be gathered so that an informed decision can be made regarding permanent changes in the system.

Closer analysis of the data shows that the error rate is one per 1,000 over a 20-month period and that the error rate is higher in some months and lower in others. Exhibit 4.9 displays the approximate order flow at this point.

The error rate per 1,000 orders is as follows, tabulated by month:

Month	Error Rate per 1,000	Month	Error Rate per 1,000
June	2.1	May	1.1
July	0.4	June	0.3
August	0.6	July	1.3
September	1.7	August	1.5
October	0.4	September	1.3
November	0.5	October	1.2
December	0.0	November	0.5
January	1.0	December	1.2
February	0.2	January	0.6
March	1.4	**Average**	**1.0**
April	2.1	**Standard Deviation**	**0.8**

Exhibit 4.9: Pharmacy Order, Initial Model

The tabulated data show that the average error rate is 1 error per 1,000 orders; the standard deviation is found to be 0.8 per 1,000 orders. These are easily calculated with any spreadsheet application. For example, the built-in Microsoft Excel functions are AVERAGE(. . .) and STDEV.P(. . .).

A histogram of the data helps to visualize what is going on. The histogram in exhibit 4.10 presents the data in a particular graphical form that shows the frequency with which each error rate occurs. The x-axis is divided into conveniently small steps. For example, in this exhibit, the step size is one-tenth of an error per 1,000. Bigger or smaller steps can be tried until a reasonable graph presents itself.

Exhibit 4.10: Histogram of Pharmacy Order

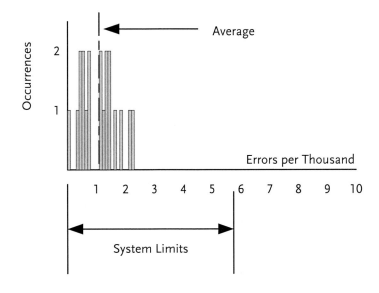

The average rate of occurrence is one per 1,000, which we already knew, and some bunching of the data appears near the average value, which seems to be reasonable. The maximum observed error rate is between two errors and three errors per 1,000; an observer would be tempted to say that somehow allowing for three errors per 1,000 would sufficiently cover the situation.

However, because the number of observations is small, it is necessary to allow for a higher error rate to cover the range of fluctuations that happen with a normal distribution. That is where Six Sigma comes in. System limits will be drawn at plus and minus six standard deviations. The lower system limit is set at zero because errors cannot occur a negative number of times. The upper system limit is set six standard deviations above the average, which comes to 5.8 errors per 1,000. With these system limits, which include an allowance for process drift, the likelihood of exceeding the upper limit is not greater than 3.4 per million.

What does this mean? This means that the present pharmacy order process cannot be relied on to have an error rate of less than 5.8 per 1,000 orders. Thus, the situation is worse than management originally thought. True, the average error rate is 1 per 1,000, but the error rate may rise as high as 5.8 per 1,000 just from random fluctuations plus an allowance for process drift. Management actions are in order.

First, the stop-gap measure of additional checking would be continued indefinitely. Second, the standard treatment schedule would be changed to allow extra time to get a replacement pharmacy order filled on an expedited basis for those cases in which the rechecking turns up an error in the pharmacy order.

The revised flow chart might look something like exhibit 4.11.

Exhibit 4.11: Revised Pharmacy Order Model

With the stop-gap procedure in place, management could set about studying and changing the system to reduce both the average error rate and the variation in error rate, considering such system changes as penmanship lessons, computer-terminal order entry, computer cross-checking for standard dosages, and computer cross-checking against the patient record. One or more of these steps would be tested on a trial basis, and when a successful system change is found and validated, the organization would ideally switch over to the better system.

UNDERSTANDING THE BASELINE

When a target process is selected, the first step to take is to gather information about how the system works currently in and around this target. This becomes the baseline against which future changes can be measured.

For the work done by the target activity or activities, are average completion times and standard deviations known? Have process control limits been calculated? Are completion times tracked? What happens if the work is done incorrectly and has to be repeated? How does that show up in the tracking record?

Every process—every system—has some variability. A key to applying Six Sigma is to *accept* that the process has some variability; this variability is a characteristic of the process and cannot be removed or reduced without changing the nature of the process. Attempting to reduce the variability by interceding in the process will only increase the variability.

In a factory, the speed of the machines determines capacity. In a service organization, management is tempted to believe that more can be done if people would just work harder, pay more attention, think ahead, hurry up, or follow orders more diligently. We do not expect machines to work faster, but we do expect humans to work faster—with no limit. This is not rational, but it seems to be true.

However, the employees are probably working about as productively as they can in the current system. Maybe a hurry-up campaign will work, briefly, once in a while, but no sustained result is likely to flow from hurry-up exhortation.

It is more useful—and part of the Six Sigma concept—to start with the view that each employee is working productively and that, if an employee is slow or making errors, he or she may need additional training or a different work setup. Straightforward analysis and corrective action on the local level is the best way to solve the particular problem and build a platform for the future.

What type of analysis is likely to help? We will now take a look at some useful tools.

PROCESS FLOW DIAGRAMS

A process flow diagram is a chart that helps management understand what is going on; it may also help participants from diverse departments to understand what is going on. The chart may even help the knowledgeable participants to understand more fully what is going on because they may never have thought about things in just the way they were presented in the chart.

Process flow charts can get out of hand very quickly if the level of detail is not adjusted to a productive level. It is better to have a family of charts than to put everything onto one. These are sometimes called the "50,000-foot view," the "1,000-foot view," and the "10-foot view."

Exhibit 4.12 shows a process flow chart for the X-ray patient described above.

Exhibit 4.12: X-Ray Visit Process Flow Chart

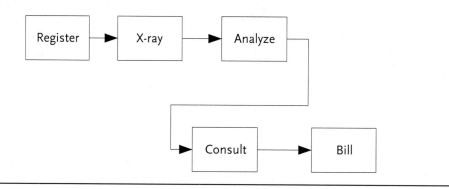

The process flow chart usually shows only the value-adding steps, not the in-between waits. For Six Sigma analysis, a process flow chart is of some value, but the time-value diagram is of more value because it gets to the heart of a key issue. The process flow chart may be thought of as an introductory chart to get to the time-value chart.

Process flow charts are easily produced by such computer applications as Visio and SmartDraw. They can also be drawn, albeit with more effort, directly in a word-processing document or spreadsheet using the primitive textbox and arrow-drawing tools provided by the application.

CONTROL CHARTS

Consider the data in exhibit 4.13, which will represent the delivery times of X-ray results over the course of a calendar week.

Exhibit 4.13: Histogram of Seven Days of Data

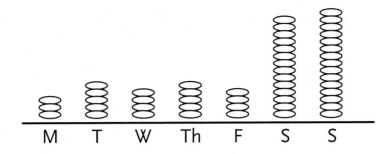

Clearly some different activity is transpiring on Saturday and Sunday; this is a system issue. Exhortation is not likely to improve weekend performance much, because a mismatch is likely between workload and staff hours or staff skills. More legwork is in order to gain a better understanding of the problem.

Look now at the variability during the Monday through Friday period. The count is not uniform: It is three, five, four, five, and four, respectively. This is the inherent variability of the process. This is what the system can do and does today. The variability is not very great—only one or two counts from day to day—but it is not zero; some variability is inherent in the daily level.

The counts are characterized by a *chronic* variability level, which is three to five units per day in the case at hand, and an *episodic* level that occurs on Saturday and Sunday, which is an additional count of about six units per day.

Suppose on a Monday the count is two. Does that show improvement? Suppose on the following day, a Tuesday, the count is six. Does that show a collapse in the system? In both cases, the answer is no. A count of two or six once in a while can be expected because of the inherent, chronic variability in the process.

Here is how to figure out what the limits on reasonable expectations are for the chronic variability in the process:

1. Ignore the weekend data and consider only the weekday data, where the chronic variability is easy to see.
2. Using a computer spreadsheet application, enter the weekday data and use the built-in functions to calculate the average value and the standard deviation of the data set. In Excel, the functions are AVERAGE(. . .) and STDEV.P(. . .). Other spreadsheet products might have slightly different names for these functions, but they all have them.

Here is how the spreadsheet should look:

Day	Count
Monday	3
Tuesday	5
Wednesday	4
Thursday	5
Friday	4
Average	4.2
Standard deviation	0.84
Three times the standard deviation	2.51

Having a simple, graphic way of knowing what process variation is to be expected is useful. This can be done by drawing lines at the average plus/minus three standard deviations levels because a normal distribution stays within plus/minus three standard deviations 99.7 percent of the time. Data points may show up outside these limits, but they are so unlikely that they deserve special scrutiny every time. If the data points stay within these limits, everything can be considered to be working the way it is expected to work given the system as it currently exists.

These limits are process control limits (see pages 45–46), even though no particular control is being applied:

Upper control limit = Average + Three standard deviations
Lower control limit = Average – Three standard deviations

Variations that fall within this control band can be considered normal variations. Variations that fall outside this band can be considered abnormal, and they call for special attention. They are probably *not* naturally occurring.

This can be monitored simply by creating a process control chart, which has the ongoing results and two lines showing the upper and lower control limit lines. The process control chart shown above would look like exhibit 4.14.

A quick look at this process control chart tells us that something odd is going on over the weekend. We already knew that, so it is comforting that the analysis confirms it.

So far, the weekend data have been considered as departures from the nominal system. However, if these data must be included because there is no way to deal with them using separate management policies or other distinct actions, the analysis would need to include all seven days of data.

Exhibit 4.14: Process Control Chart Based on Five Days' Operations

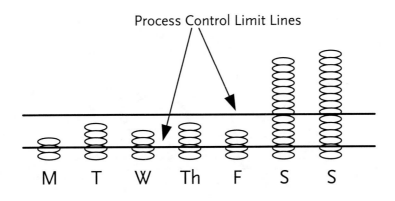

Process Control Limit Lines

M T W Th F S S

Repeat the Excel spreadsheet calculations to include seven days of data:

Day	Count
Monday	3
Tuesday	5
Wednesday	4
Thursday	5
Friday	4
Saturday	14
Sunday	15
Average	7.14
Standard deviation	5.08
Three times the standard deviation	15.24

In this case, the lower control chart limit is negative, which has no physical meaning and can be set to zero (see exhibit 4.15). This happens because the normal distribution, used for convenience, is not the perfect representation of the data. However, little practical benefit comes from searching for a better representation in most real cases.

Including the weekend data makes a big difference in both the average value and the standard deviation. As shown in the two tables above, the standard deviation estimate changed from 0.84 to 5.08, a change of 4.24 units. The wider process control band now encompasses all of the data points on the diagram because all of the points have been accepted as normal points.

Exhibit 4.15: Process Control Chart Based on Seven Days' Operations

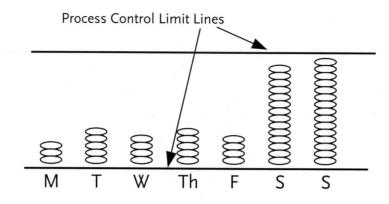

The name for this kind of chart, "process control chart," may give the impression that something is being controlled and that the data points are being forced to stay within the control band; this is not the case. The process control limits are characteristics of the process as it presently exists. Nothing is being controlled in the usual meaning of the word.

The value of the process control limits is that any data point falling outside the control band is an unusual data point (one that would occur only about once per 1,000 events) if the process that is being tracked is still running the way it was when the process control lines were drawn. Any point outside the lines may be all right, but chances are something exceptional is happening. Any point outside the process control limit lines should get close scrutiny. Furthermore, if a pattern develops in which several points fall outside the lines, the process has changed and something is wrong.

For this tracking purpose alone, the process control chart makes good practice for every process in the system that impinges on service. These charts are easy to make and easy to understand, and they have direct meaning for service management.

SIX SIGMA SYSTEM LIMIT LINES

In addition to the process control lines, Six Sigma adds two more lines: the system limit lines. The space between the system limit lines is called the system limit band. The system limit lines are drawn six standard deviations away from the process average, so the system limit band is twice as wide as the process control band. Six

Sigma also requires that the process average be no closer to either system limit than 4.5 times the process average value; this may happen if the process drifts or is changed in some way. Normal process variability will produce points outside the system limits only a few times in a million events.

The system limits constitute a conceptual fence between this process and the overall system. The process agrees to keep itself within the system limits, and the system agrees not to demand anything from the system beyond staying within the system limits. If the organization wants more performance from this process, some change has to be made to improve the process so that the system limit band can be contracted.

THE MANAGEMENT INTEREST

Note that the level of management interest is different for the process control limits and the system limits. The process control limits may be seen as a matter of local, process-management interest. If data points show up that are outside the process control band or if some trend shows up within the process control band, local management will want to step in to find out what has changed in the process to cause this deviant behavior.

The system limits are a matter of interest to higher management because the interfaces between operating departments are represented by the system limits. Local initiatives to improve the process may be offered up to the organization as proposed tightening of the system limits. On the other hand, the local management can defend the present system limits on the process by producing process control charts and asserting that that is the way things are and that the system limits can only be changed if measures are taken to improve the process itself.

To take the simple example above, we will start with the chart that is based on all seven days of performance (exhibit 4.15). Local management can say that the present system, which has poor performance on weekends, requires that the system limits be set at a high level, as is shown in the control chart in exhibit 4.16. The upper system limit is at 38 units, and the lower system limit is at zero. No points appear anywhere near the upper system limit. That is to be expected, for only a few points in a million would approach this limit, and with only seven daily total samples on this chart, few-in-a-million events are not likely.

Should the system limit be drawn at a lower level, thereby soaking up the white space between the process control limit and the upper system limit? That can only be done at the risk that data points will impinge on the system limit just through normal process fluctuation much more often than a few times in a million. Given

Exhibit 4.16: Control Chart with System Limits

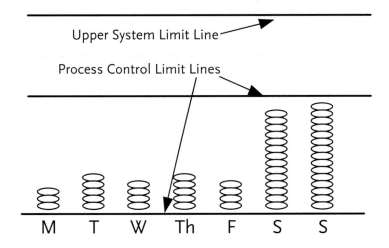

that the whole point of Six Sigma is to prevent that, Six Sigma policy is to leave the upper system limit alone.

Now, the charts draw attention to the weekend data. If something were done differently on the weekends, that would constitute a *change in the process*. If the steps bring the weekend data down to about the level of the weekday points, the process control limits and the system limits can be redrawn after a suitable trial period. The contraction of the system limits could then be used as a basis to revise the interface with the neighboring operating unit and to improve overall system performance.

DATA TRACKING

Track the process by plotting data points as they happen on a process control chart. Set the process control limits by calculating the average value and the standard deviation of the samples in hand. If the sample count is lower than 20, redo the calculations when 20 samples are in hand. Over time, redo the calculations about once a month.

Examine the process control chart; that is the point of creating it in the first place. Are the plotted points within the control band? Are the plotted points balanced around the average? Are the plotted points showing a periodic pattern? Are the plotted points drifting away from the average?

We will now look at the tracking of data on a typical process control chart, as shown in exhibit 4.17.

Exhibit 4.17: Typical Tracking Chart

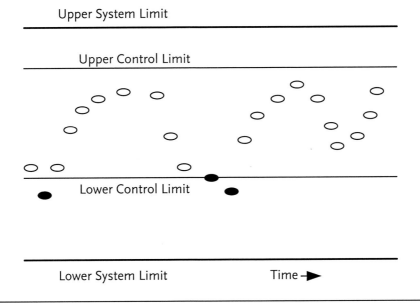

Upper System Limit

Upper Control Limit

Lower Control Limit

Lower System Limit   Time ➤

Are there exceptional points that call for further attention?

This chart shows one point right on the process control lower limit and two points below the process control lower limit (highlighted as black dots on the chart). In this case, at least two and probably three points merit special attention, and some legwork is in order to see if it can be determined what was different on those two or three occasions. It cannot be ruled out that these are just naturally occurring points from the distribution, but they look odd and should be checked out.

Now look at the rest of the points, which show a pronounced cyclical pattern. Cyclical patterns are common enough, often following day/night or early-in-shift/late-in-shift patterns. The fact that there is a cyclical pattern is not necessarily a concern, but it is something that might bear a little further study. Perhaps the process could be changed to reduce the swing over the cycle, such as by retraining or getting equipment tuned up before the shift starts. If the cyclic swing could be cut in half, both the process control limit band and the system limit band could be cut about in half, too, which would lead in general to an improvement in the overall system performance.

Note that the process control band is not centered between the system limits. This should be marked for eventual consideration, even if the present ratios meet the Six Sigma design rules.

We will now consider another tracking example.

Exhibit 4.18: Process Tracking with Drift

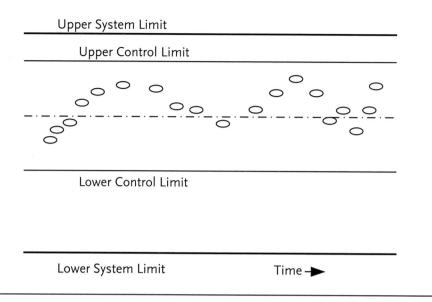

Exhibit 4.18 is a similar plot to the previous chart, but note that here all of the points are within the process control band. The cyclical pattern appears again, and there now seems to be a bit of an upward drift, too. It looks like the bottom points are moving up more than the top points, so the average may be shifting upward. This hypothesis can be tested by tracking the average separately (as will be considered next), but for the time being, we will look at what this chart shows.

The process is believed to be following a normal distribution, and because the normal distribution is symmetric with regard to its average value, half the points should be below the average line, and half should be above. What are the odds that the next point will be above the average? One in two. What are the odds that the next two points will be above the average? One in four. The next three points? One in eight. The next four points? One in 16. The next five points? One in 32. The next ten points above the line? Less than one in 1,000. So, if several points in a row (or nearly all of several points in a row) fall on one side of the average, the process has probably somehow changed and some unknown event is currently causing this to happen. Now would be a good time to look into the matter, before the process drifts so far that the system limits are in jeopardy.

MANAGEMENT VIEW OF MULTISTEP PROCESSES

The average yield of a multistep process is the product of the average yields of the individual steps. The average duration of a multistep process is the sum of the average durations of the individual steps. The standard deviations add like the sides of triangles, by taking the square root of the sum of the squares.

We now consider a four-step process with yields and durations as shown in this table:

Stage	Yield	Standard Deviation Yield	Duration (Hours)	Standard Deviation Duration (Hours)
1	99%	1%	2	0.3
2	95%	2%	12	1.5
3	95%	2%	8	0.5
4	94%	4%	1	0.1
Combined	84%	5%	23	1.6

Looking at each step individually shows that the yields, although not particularly good, do not look particularly bad. Combined, they look pretty bad. If only 84 percent of patients are getting their treatment right the first time all the way through, that means that 16 percent, on average, are being held up for additional treatment or to fix paperwork or something else unplanned. On first approximation, 16 percent of the organization's effort is going toward rework.

Suppose we calculate control limits and system limits on the four-step process:

	Yield	Duration (Hours)
Control Limits		
Upper	99%	27.8
Lower	69%	18.2
System Limits		
Upper	100%	32.7
Lower	54%	13.3

The control limits are approached a few times per 1,000, so the organization can expect to see as few as 69 percent of any group of patients flowing through the system with no error and, consequently, as many as 31 percent of any group of patients being held up for rework. The organization can expect to see treatment durations ranging from 18 to 28 hours.

On a conservative planning basis, management would use the system limit values, planning on a contingency basis to see yields as low as 54 percent for any group of patients and durations as high as 33 hours. Management may elect to study more closely those cases that flow through the system very quickly. There is something favorable about these. Are they a peculiar group of people? Are they being treated in some particular way that others are not? Is something here to be learned that might apply to the population as a whole?

Management can also study the least favorable of these cases to see what is going wrong. The bad cases get management attention because a clamor for attention will likely be raised by the patient group, by the department managers who are seeing their work backed up, and by employees who find themselves doing work twice. It takes more management willpower to look into the favorable cases because clamor is not likely, and yet it is in studying the favorable cases that a new lesson may be learned.

QUANTITATIVE PROCESS ANALYSIS

We will now look a little more closely at the quantitative methods that support Six Sigma analysis. Nothing in this section requires any higher mathematics training; all arithmetic will be presented on the basis that the reader has convenient access to a computer and a spreadsheet application. The specifics here will follow Microsoft Excel nomenclature; all spreadsheets have these same functions, although they may have slightly different names and arrangements of arguments.

We want to estimate the average and standard deviation of observed values. If lots of data are in hand, getting sufficient estimates of these two parameters is very easy by using the spreadsheet functions AVERAGE(. . .) and STDEV.P(. . .). These can be applied to prior data to characterize the process baseline, and they can be applied during a trial to characterize the effect of the changes introduced for the purposes of the trial.

In health service processes, often relatively few data are on hand, and the rate of generating new data is rather slow. Therefore, it is often necessary to consider methods that apply to sparse data sets.

When the data sets are "rich" in number, the process average value and the process standard deviation can be tracked directly, as will be shown shortly. When the data sets are sparse, indirect methods will be developed and applied.

TRACKING THE PROCESS

Plotting data points directly on a process control chart, with process limit lines at plus and minus three standard deviations and with system limits at plus and minus six standard deviations, is good practice. Points that fall outside of the process control limits are points worthy of attention every time because this should happen only a few times per 1,000. Consider these as early warnings. Points that fall outside the system limit lines are a cause for alarm because this should happen only a few times per million and will likely upset operations beyond the immediate operating unit.

If a great many data points are being generated, it may be appropriate to plot just a sample of the total data set using some rule to decide which to plot and which not to plot. Getting the sampling plan right takes some thought, and this matter will be covered in detail in case 13. Also, if there are a lot of data, it may be helpful to aggregate the data into subsets, perhaps by department or by shift, and to plot just the subset averages and subset standard deviations. This is particularly the case for the subset averages; Six Sigma makes a special allowance for drift in the average, so observing whether any drifting is taking place is helpful.

TRACKING THE PROCESS AVERAGE DIRECTLY

Set the rule for dividing up the data into subsets, perhaps by shift or by department. Calculate the average value of each subset using AVERAGE(. . .). Plot the results on a tracking plot (see exhibit 4.19). This plot is often called an *X-bar plot*, because it uses the X-bar to denote the subset averages.

If plotted on the same scale used for plotting individual data points, the X-bar points will show a much tighter pattern than the individual data points; this is reasonable because the average will move around a lot less than will individual samples.

It may be helpful to plot limit lines at 1.5 standard deviations from the established average. Six Sigma makes allowance for drift in the process average value of as much as 1.5 standard deviations. If the average shows signs of

Exhibit 4.19: Tracking Chart for Sample Averages

violating this allowance, it is time to pay special attention to the process to see what's going on.

It is often useful to develop process control limits for the X-bar values and to take these X-bar values as a new population. (It is a source of endless confusion that the X-bar population has its own standard deviation, which is different and distinct from the standard deviation of the underlying population. It is a good thing it does, though, because this is the basis for the central limit theorem, which will be covered in case 12 and is the reason that the normal distribution is so popular in everyday statistical analysis.) Using the X-bar values, apply STDEV.P(. . .) and plot lines at plus and minus three times this value from the established process average value. If the process is well-behaved, the X-bar points will fall within these control limits except for a few times in 1,000. This is an early warning line.

The observation technique is the same. Are there exceptional points? Is there cyclic behavior? Is there drift?

TRACKING THE PROCESS STANDARD DEVIATION DIRECTLY

To track the process standard deviation directly, the method is the same. First, set a rule for dividing the sample data into subsets, perhaps by shift or department. For each set, calculate the standard deviation within that set using STDEV.P(. . .). Plot the points; this is often called an *S-plot*.

If the STDEV.P(. . .) values are collected, they form a new population that has an average value and a standard deviation all its own. These parameters can be used to make a new control chart with limit lines at plus and minus three times the standard deviation of this new population. If points on this control chart approach these limit lines more than a few times per 1,000, it is time to pay attention. These are early warning lines.

DEALING WITH SPARSE DATA SETS

If the number of samples in the total available population is lower than about 20, the AVERAGE(. . .) and STDEV.P(. . .) functions will produce results, but these results will be uncertain. The same is true for any subset with fewer than about 20 samples.

Some methods for dealing with these sparse data sets do not eliminate the uncertainty (that would be impossible), but they do have the merit of telling you what that uncertainty is. These methods generate *confidence intervals*, which are bands within which the underlying population's average value and, separately, the underlying population's standard deviation are likely to fall for a given confidence level. The confidence level is stipulated by the analyst; it is typically 75 or 90 percent, occasionally 95 or 99 percent, or, sometimes just for fun, 99.9 percent.

Before getting into the arithmetic, let us perform the following mental exercise. Suppose there are 25 people in a room, and their average age is calculated down to the day. For this example, the age will be 27 years and 87 days. Now, if we take a sample of five people from that same group and calculate their average age, would we expect to get 27 years and 87 days? No; we would expect to get some other average for this small subgroup. Suppose we increase the sample size to ten people and calculate the average age of this group. We would not expect to get 27 years and 87 days, but we could expect to get closer to that because the sample is larger. Suppose we took a sample of 20. Intuitively we would expect to be getting a very good estimate of the real average number.

Student

Modern applied statistics began in 1908 with the publication of "The Probable Error of a Mean" by William Sealy Gosset, who was using the nom de plume "Student" (Student 1908). Gosset was a brewer for Guinness Breweries and an amateur mathematician.

Now, rather than expecting to get the right answer, suppose we ask only that we get *close to* the right answer. Suppose we ask that we get within 30 days of the right answer, or 60 days, or 90 days. If some cost is involved in getting each value, we might do a trade-off between cost and precision of result; this would also cause us to consider just how much precision we really need in the answer.

Suppose we now say that we want to know how confident we can be that the answer is really within our stipulated range of, say, 30 days. Can we be 100 percent confident? 95 percent confident? 75 percent confident? 50 percent confident? If we are betting that the right answer is within the specified range, what odds do we want to take that the right answer is within this range?

When we deal with sparse data, we make estimates of the average value and standard deviation, and these estimates are intervals. We combine a confidence level and a sample size, and we compute the interval. The higher the confidence level we set, the wider the interval; the smaller the sample size, the wider the interval. A wide interval may be worthless to us, so we set about gathering more data to increase the sample size and thereby reduce the interval size.

A high degree of confidence in the outcome is not always needed, and in these cases a lower confidence level can be used and a smaller interval computed. We will be wrong more often, but we will know that when we set the confidence level.

Two statistical methods will be applied when using the Six Sigma process. For the confidence intervals for the population average value, the Student's t-method and distribution are applied. For the confidence intervals for the population standard deviation, the chi-square (the *chi* sound is hard, as in "chiropractor") method and distribution will be applied.

These methods are easy enough to apply if a spreadsheet is available to do the arithmetic. The method is shown in the next section, and tables of results covering the usual range of interest are also provided. If you are performing the analysis using a spreadsheet, you can follow the method given here. If you are computing the analysis by hand, just use the tabulated results shown.

If these methods are applied to rich populations (those with a lot of sample values), they will yield a confidence interval that is only a little larger than a point; they do not provide any useful information if there is hardly any uncertainty in the calculations. Therefore, for rich populations, confidence intervals are not worth the bother.

CONFIDENCE INTERVALS FOR THE POPULATION AVERAGE VALUE

Proceed as follows:

1. Select the sample set to be analyzed and note the number of samples.
2. Compute the set average and standard deviation using AVERAGE(. . .) and STDEV.P(. . .).

3. Select a confidence level such as 90 percent.
4. Compute the inverse Student t-factor by T.INV(100 percent minus the confidence level, number of samples). For example, you would enter T.INV(100% – 90%, 15) for a confidence level of 90 percent and a sample size of 15. Call the result t'.
5. Multiply the STDEV.P(. . .) value by t'. Add this to the AVERAGE(. . .) result to get the upper limit on the confidence interval, and subtract the same from the AVERAGE(. . .) value to get the lower limit on the confidence interval.
6. If this is being applied to subsets, plotting the intervals can be instructive.

Here is a quick example:

Calculating Confidence Intervals for the Average: Spreadsheet Method	
Count	15
Confidence level	90%
T.INV(100% – confidence level, number of samples)	1.753
Sample average value	12.7
Sample standard deviation	1.8
Confidence interval, upper limit	15.86
Confidence interval, lower limit	9.54

The meaning of confidence interval is this: The likelihood that the true value lies within this interval is equal to the asserted confidence level. So, if the asserted confidence level is 90 percent, the likelihood is 90 percent that the confidence interval covers the true value. The converse is also true: If the confidence level is 90 percent, there is a 10 percent chance that the true value is *not* covered by the interval. If this is done repeatedly over time, the confidence intervals will be seen to cover the true value about as often as would be expected from the confidence level asserted.

Consider exhibit 4.20, which shows 20 confidence intervals computed in this way for a 75 percent confidence level and sample sizes of ten. These are all drawn from a normal distribution having an average value of zero. One would expect that about three-quarters of the confidence intervals would cover the zero line. Fifteen of them do, and two others come close, so this is about as expected. Even so, three of the intervals seem to be quite far away from the zero line, and if it were the analyst's bad luck to draw these, the analyst could be led astray.

As more data come to hand, the uncertainty can be reduced by including the additional data points in the analysis. If all 200 of the points used to plot these

Exhibit 4.20: Tracking Chart for Confidence Intervals on the Average Value

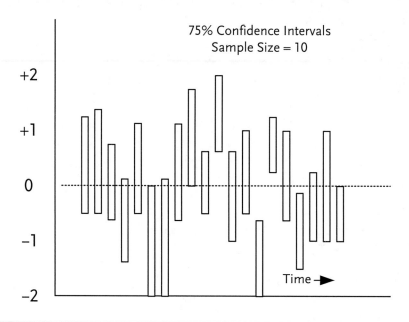

confidence intervals were used to calculate the average, the result would be a confidence interval of 0.08, which is pretty close to zero. This shows that using sparse-data analysis, including confidence intervals, while a larger data set is being gathered, can be useful. Even with the inherent uncertainty, some information, properly interpreted, is better than none.

The next table shows the multipliers to use when calculating the confidence intervals on the average value for a range commonly of interest. Select an entry from the table, multiply the selected entry by the sample standard deviation found by STDEV.P(. . .), and then add the product to (subtract the product from) the sample average value found by AVERAGE(. . .) to get the upper (lower) confidence interval limit on the average value of the underlying population.

Multipliers for Average Value Confidence Intervals

Count	50% Confidence	75% Confidence	90% Confidence
5	0.727	1.301	2.015
10	0.700	1.221	1.812
15	0.691	1.197	1.753
20	0.687	1.185	1.725

To do the same example from above, using the table instead of the spreadsheet formula, you would proceed as follows:

Calculating Confidence Intervals for the Average: Tabulated Values Method	
Count	15
Confidence level	90%
t-value from table for this count and confidence level	1.753
Sample average value	12.7
Sample standard deviation	1.8
Confidence interval, upper limit	15.86
Confidence interval, lower limit	9.54

CONFIDENCE INTERVALS FOR THE POPULATION STANDARD DEVIATION

The logic for using confidence intervals rather than point values is the same for the population standard deviation as it is for the population average value. If the data set is sparse, using a confidence interval yields better results than believing the point value provided by STDEV.P(. . .). Indeed, using confidence intervals for the standard deviation is even more appropriate because the standard deviation settles down more slowly as the sample count increases than the average value does. The mechanics for both, however, are nearly the same. The chi-square method and distribution are used to compute the confidence interval for the standard deviation. The steps are as follows:

1. Note the sample set size—say 15.
2. Select a confidence level—say 75 percent. Select two limits, the difference between which equals the confidence level—say 87.5 percent and 12.5 percent.
3. For each of these, compute the chi-square factor by applying CHIINV(upper limit, set count less one)—for our example, CHIINV(87.5%, 14). Repeat for the lower limit—CHIINV(12.5%, 14).
4. Calculate the upper multiplier by taking the square root of the ratio of (sample count less one) over the upper chi-square factor from step 3—in this case, SQRT[14/CHIINV(87.5%, 14)]. Repeat using the lower limit to get the lower multiplier—in this case, SQRT[14/CHIINV(12.5%, 14)].
5. Compute the set standard deviation with STDEV.P(. . .).

6. Multiply the set standard deviation by the upper multiplier to get the upper end of the confidence interval. Repeat using the lower multiplier to get the lower end of the confidence interval. Doing this all at once, the upper limit would be, for this example, STDEV.P(. . .) × SQRT[14/CHIINV(14, 87.5%)], and the lower limit would be, for this example, STDEV.P(. . .) × SQRT[14/CHIINV(4, 12.5%)].

Note that the set average value plays no part in the calculation of the confidence interval for the standard deviation.

Here is an example worked out:

Calculating Confidence Intervals for the Standard Deviation: Spreadsheet Method

Count	15
Confidence level	75%
Upper cutoff	87.5%
Lower cutoff	12.5%
Chi-square factor, upper	8.266
Chi-square factor, lower	20.166
Upper multiplier	1.301
Lower multiplier	0.833
Sample standard deviation, taken from example above	1.8
Upper confidence interval limit on standard deviation	2.343
Lower confidence interval limit on standard deviation	1.500

This arithmetic is easy enough for a spreadsheet to do, but it is exactly the sort of step-by-step arithmetic that invites trouble when done by hand. To keep the by-hand analyst out of trouble, the following table skips all of the arithmetic and just gives the multipliers to be applied to the sample standard deviation for a useful range of confidence levels and sample sizes.

Multipliers to Apply to the Sample Standard Deviation

Sample Count	50% Confidence		75% Confidence		90% Confidence	
	Lower	Upper	Lower	Upper	Lower	Upper
5	0.862	1.442	0.745	1.812	0.649	2.372
10	0.889	1.235	0.804	1.413	0.729	1.645
15	0.904	1.174	0.833	1.301	0.769	1.460
20	0.915	1.142	0.852	1.246	0.794	1.370

These multipliers get applied to the sample standard deviation to get the upper and lower limits on the confidence interval for the population's standard deviation.

Here is the same example, worked from the table:

Calculating Confidence Intervals for the Standard Deviation: Tabulated Values Method	
Count	15
Confidence level	75%
Upper multiplier from table	1.301
Lower multiplier from table	0.833
Sample standard deviation, taken from example above	1.8
Upper confidence interval limit on standard deviation	2.343
Lower confidence interval limit on standard deviation	1.500

Note that the upper and lower multipliers are not equal; this is because the chi-square distribution is not symmetric.

Exhibit 4.21 shows some confidence intervals on the population standard deviation with various confidence level requirements and sample sizes. The samples are drawn from a normal distribution with standard deviation equal to unity.

For the sample count of two, the 90 percent and 75 percent confidence bars are truncated at the upper end to keep them in the chart. The actual numbers are about

Exhibit 4.21: Effect of Sample Count on Standard Deviation Confidence Interval Size

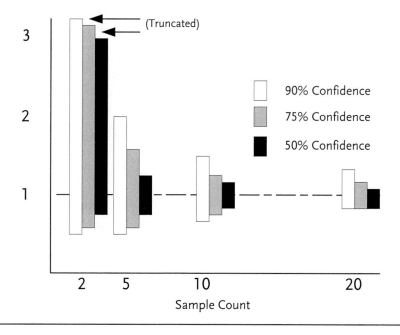

15 and 6, which means that the bars are so long as to be worthless for estimating where the underlying standard deviation might be.

Each of the bars represents a confidence interval, and the longer the bar, the less helpful the estimate. To put it more positively, a smaller bar provides a more helpful estimate.

A 50 percent confidence factor is the lowest confidence factor worth the bother. A 75 percent confidence factor is reasonable for general tracking of sample data, and a confidence factor of 90 or 95 percent should be held for those applications where there are plenty of sample points and the significance of the result is great.

To confirm that the behavior of confidence intervals on the population's standard deviation follows the behavior of confidence intervals on the population's average value, exhibit 4.22 shows a chart displaying 20 different confidence intervals computed by taking samples from the same normal distribution having a true standard deviation of 2.00.

Exhibit 4.22: Tracking Chart for Confidence Intervals for the Standard Deviation

Because the asserted confidence level is 75 percent, one would expect about three-quarters of the confidence intervals to cover the true value, which is the 2.00 line. Four of the confidence intervals do not cover the 2.00 line, and a couple of the others appear to just touch it; that would seem to be consistent with a 75 percent confidence interval, by definition, because about three-quarters of the intervals cover the known and true standard deviation.

With all 200 data points in hand (using all 20 of the sets of 10 samples), applying STDEV.P(. . .) returns a point estimate for the population's standard deviation of 1.996. Compare that with the true value of 2.00. Once again, having plenty of data points reduces uncertainty and allows the analyst to skip the bother of calculating confidence intervals.

The application of the confidence interval to the population standard deviation for sparse data sets is this: Use the confidence interval cautiously until more data points come to light. Having an estimate, even with uncertainty, is better than having no information at all. Using STDEV.P(. . .) to do a point estimate of the population standard deviation with a sparse data set is rash.

REPEATABILITY AND REPRODUCIBILITY

Employee teams repeat tasks. The extent to which the outcomes are about the same, time after time, is called *repeatability*. Different employee teams also perform these same tasks. The extent to which the second group has outcomes that are about the same as those of the first group is called *reproducibility*. Repeatability and reproducibility are interesting to isolate because different actions are required to improve each one.

This analysis is traditionally called *gauge analysis* because the original question was, "How variable are worker A's readings of a certain gauge, and how much difference does it make if worker B reads the gauge instead?" With digital gauges these days, that issue has largely gone away. However, for other tasks, the issue is still germane. For instance, it may be of interest to compare the results of work done on different shifts, work done by novices versus that done by experienced staff, winter versus summer work, hot day versus cold day results, or any other discriminating parameter.

Suppose data are available for the outcomes of a task, and suppose it is known which tasks were done by group A and which were done by group B. We wish to know if any significant difference is found between the two groups.

Proceed as follows:

Calculate the average values and standard deviations for subset A and subset B using AVERAGE(. . .) and STDEV.P(. . .). If they look to be about the same, operate on the basis that they *are* the same (that no distinction exists between group A and group B), at least until more data come to hand.

If they look to be somewhat different, take guidance from the following table:

Sample Count	Difference	Action
~ 100 or more	Large	Believe the values
	Small	Believe the values
~ 50 or so	Large	Believe the direction
	Small	Believe no change
~ 25 or so	Large	Do confidence test
	Small	Believe no change
~ 10 or so	Large	Get more data
	Small	Get more data

The confidence tests, which will now be described, can be applied to any sample size. However, for large sample sizes, the result will just confirm what direct observation has already told you, and for tiny sample sizes, the result will not give you much guidance. For middle-size samples, doing some simple analysis is worthwhile if only to help decide whether to try to get more data so that more precision can be obtained in the analysis.

Step 1. Are the average values different? Use the following test to see if the underlying populations have the same average value.

Tabulate the sample subsets in a spreadsheet.

Apply the built-in spreadsheet function T.TEST(first sample set, second sample set); T.TEST is the Excel function that uses the Student's t-function to calculate the probabilities. The value returned by T.TEST is a probability that the means of the two underlying populations are the same—in this case, say 67 percent.

This test is certainly easy to perform, but it is very sensitive to small changes in the sample data. Such changes, which may be hardly noticeable to the analyst, might cause the result to change from 66 to 50 percent, so caution is in order. To see the sensitivity, consider four sets of 25 data points all drawn from the same underlying population. Because the underlying population is the same, the "right answer" is a high confidence that each pair are the same. The question at hand is, does the T.TEST analysis give the high-confidence answer?

Set Pair	Confidence Factor That the Sets Save the Same Average Value
A-B	95%
A-C	81%
A-D	97%
B-C	74%
B-D	99%
C-D	76%

Some of these pairs show high confidence that they have the same mean, but for one pair, B-C, the confidence level is rather modest at 74 percent, and for another pair, C-D, the confidence level is only slightly better at 76 percent. In the normal course of events, the analyst would not have four sets but only two, and knowing that the results may depend on chance, the analyst will proceed with some caution.

The next question is what to do with the answer. If the answer is 93 percent, the test may be helpful because it would reveal that the two populations very likely have the same average value. If the answer is 4 percent, the test may be helpful because it is saying that the two populations very likely do *not* have the same average value. If the answer is 43, 55, or 68 percent, you're stuck. More data are needed.

Step 2. Are the standard deviations different? Tabulate the sample subsets in a spreadsheet.

Apply the built-in function F.TEST(first sample set, second sample set). F.TEST is the Excel function using the F distribution to calculate the probabilities. The function returns, say, 45 percent.

This test is also easy to perform, and like the T.TEST, it is very sensitive to small changes in the data sets and must be used cautiously. More data will always help. If the outcome is neither near one nor near zero, the test is inconclusive and more data are required.

Here is the F.TEST applied to the same four sets of 25 samples each, all drawn from the same normal distribution:

Set Pairs	Confidence That the Sets Have the Same Standard Deviation
A-B	13%
A-C	78%
A-D	37%
B-C	21%
B-D	52%
C-D	54%

This table uses exactly the same data sets as were used above to test for same/different average values. This time, the test is to find the same/different standard deviations. The answers are much worse, being neither very close to unity nor close to zero. In fact, the answers are no help at all.

This is often the case when testing for the standard deviation with modest-size samples because the standard deviation is much more volatile than the average value. The only cure is to get more data. Suspend judgment in the meantime.

ANALYSIS OF VARIANCE: REGRESSION

The *variance* of a distribution is the square of the standard deviation. It happens that variances can be added together and subtracted from one another. If there are only two variables, say length and weight, the variance of the entire set can be decomposed into a variance with length, a variance with weight, and perhaps a cross-term varying with both length and weight. Because of this, it is useful to apply this law to gain insight into the workings of the process being examined.

One common application is called *regression*, which is the fitting of a formula to fit the data set. The most common formula to fit is that of a straight line. Excel and other spreadsheets do the heavy lifting, so a few keystrokes will provide an analysis. Rather than derive formulae here, we will proceed to look at examples.

In the first case (exhibit 4.23), a straight line is fitted to a collection of points that look like a straight line using the Excel linear regression tool. The chart shows that this might be a reasonable model; this is known because we asked the spreadsheet to plot both the data and the fitted line so that the goodness of fit can be inspected by eye. This is always good practice in statistical analysis because, although the computer can do the arithmetic, the analyst has to provide the common sense. In this case, the fit appears to be reasonable, but it is not very good at the right-hand end of the data.

Exhibit 4.23: Linear Regression Example

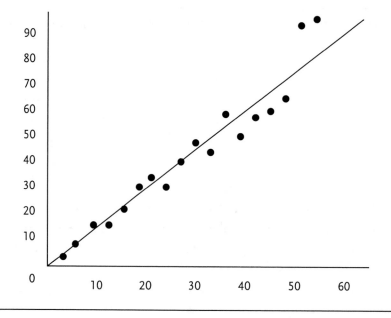

Excel not only gives the fitted parameters, it provides a lot of analysis of its work. However, as the Excel labeling is obscure, we will provide several of its labels and their hidden meaning here:

Excel Label	Meaning
ANOVA	Analysis of variance
Degrees of freedom	Degrees of freedom
SS	Sum of squares
MS	Mean of the sum of squares
F	Value from the F distribution
Significance	Goodness-of-fit value
Regression	Variability accounted for by the fit
Residual	Variability remaining after the fit
Intercept	Y value when X = 0
X variable 1	Slope of the fitted line

Excel does use additional labels and values that may be of interest in some cases. There are online tutorials on most such topics.

The degrees of freedom are related to the size of the sample set. The total number of degrees of freedom is equal to the size of the sample set. One degree of freedom is assigned in the analysis to the fit, and the rest of the degrees of freedom are assigned to the residual, which is to say the lack of fit, point by point.

The F value comes from the F distribution, and a higher value is better than a lower value. Whether the F value is high enough can be evaluated by looking at the significance value computed by Excel. In this case, a low number is good. A significance value *below* the level of interest, say 5 percent, means that the fit is good "at the 5 percent level of significance." The significance level is the complement of the confidence level; a significance level of 5 percent corresponds to a confidence level of 95 percent.

Another way of determining the goodness of fit is to look at the sum of squares (SS) value for the regression as a proportion of the total sum of squares. If the proportion is high, the fit is better than if the proportion is low. There is no numerical test for good versus bad for this parameter.

To fit a straight line to data, use the Excel function LINEST(. . .). To perform more sophisticated fits and analysis, load and activate the Analysis ToolPak by following these steps:

1. Click the File tab, click Options, and then click the Add-Ins category.
2. In the Manage box, select Excel Add-Ins and then click Go.
3. In the Add-Ins box, check the Analysis ToolPak check box, and then click OK.

With the Analysis ToolPak loaded and activated, select Data on the menu bar, then select Data Analysis from the ribbon. Select the tool of interest from the drop-down list.

Caution: Excel does not reapply these tools if the data change. So, if the data change, it is necessary to repeat the steps above to force Excel to repeat the regression analysis. Excel does not warn you about this, so be careful.

Here are the data points used to produce the regression line in exhibit 4.23:

X	Y	X	Y
2	3.57	22	27.86
4	6.23	24	42.38
6	11.97	26	33.89
8	8.27	28	51.09
10	15.02	30	37.10
12	21.97	32	39.71
14	26.02	34	46.21
16	17.03	36	46.23
18	25.58	38	51.90
20	33.44	40	78.74

Regression Analysis: Straight-Line Fit	
Result	Value
Intercept	0.23
Confidence interval on intercept, lower end	−6.63
Confidence interval on intercept, upper end	7.09
X variable 1 (slope)	1.48
Confidence interval on slope, lower end	1.19
Confidence interval on slope, upper end	1.76

The confidence intervals are calculated at a 95 percent confidence level by default.

Let us now look at the results. The confidence interval on the intercept is –6.63 to +7.09. This is a pretty wide confidence interval, so we cannot have much confidence that we know the intercept very well at all. The confidence interval for the slope is 1.19 to 1.76. This is also a little on the wide side. Both fitted parameters are only somewhat pinned down.

Look again at the fitted line and the data points in exhibit 4.23. By inspection, the fit is pretty good. Yet, as we just saw by analysis, the fit is rather uncertain; this shows that the analytic tools are awfully conservative by their very nature. However, that is the best analysis anybody knows how to do, so it is up to the analyst to consider matters and make a judgment. Using the calculated values blindly is not good practice.

As another example, consider a regression analysis of another set of data, this one showing a cyclical pattern (exhibit 4.24):

Exhibit 4.24: Linear Regression on Cyclical Data

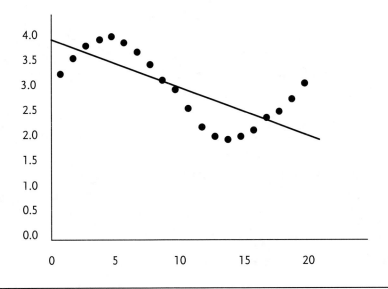

Here, the Excel regression tool has fitted a straight line, and the fitted line seems to balance points above against points below the line. However, the fit does not make any sense because a straight line is a very poor model for the data. (Hint: That is the point of this example.)

Let us see if Excel tells us that the fit does not make any sense:

Result	Value
Intercept	3.96
Confidence interval on intercept, lower end	3.48
Confidence interval on intercept, upper end	4.44
X variable 1 (slope)	−0.09
Confidence interval on slope, lower end	−0.13
Confidence interval on slope, upper end	−0.05

In this case, the confidence intervals are quite narrow. The confidence interval for the intercept is a mere 3.48 to 4.44, and the confidence interval for the slope is −0.13 to −0.05. Because both intervals are narrow, just looking at the numbers would cause the analyst to think that this straight line is a pretty good data model. However, it is not. The starting assumption—that the data can be represented by a straight line—is weak.

As with any statistical analysis, if the data sets were larger, the confidence intervals would be tighter. However, as has just been shown and can be plainly seen by looking at the fitted curve and the sample data, there is more to getting a decent fit than getting tight confidence intervals. Excel is perfectly happy to perform more complicated regressions involving more variables; the difficulty is finding some way to plot the data and the results so that some judgment can be made about the sensibility of the fitted functions. Proceed with caution. Some particular applications of multiple regression will appear later in this book.

Commercial statistical software packages include surface plotting tools that can sometimes provide a sufficient means for making a visual examination. For regression analysis going beyond one or two variables, look for a commercial package if only to get the surface plotting functionality.

To summarize:

1. To seek a relationship between variables, a regression analysis may help. Plotting the data and plotting the fitted line are absolutely necessary as part of the evaluation of the fit.
2. Visual examination of the fit is likely to be more useful than careful scrutiny of the confidence intervals or residuals or other derived statistical factors.

TIME-WEIGHTED VALUES

Statistics software packages usually offer to plot time-weighted values. However, these are not likely to be of interest in healthcare. The idea can be explained quickly enough. Start with the last several points and multiply the most recent value by one, the preceding value by a weighting factor, the value before that by the weighting factor squared, and so on. Add these up to get a weighted value, divide by the number of values used, and plot the result. Sometimes, a more complicated divisor is used, but the idea is the same. If the weighting factor is unity, this just gives a usual average of the last several data points, also known as the *boxcar average*.

If the weighting factor is less than 1, say 0.8, the more distant points are multiplied by smaller and smaller factors and contribute less and less to the final weighted value. This puts emphasis on the last point or two, and it emphasizes any lack of precision in the measurement. Because many of the data points in healthcare will be estimated and hand-recorded, they will be imprecise; therefore, emphasizing imprecise values is not likely to be helpful.

If the weighting factor is greater than 1, say 1.2, the more distant points are multiplied by greater and greater factors and contribute more and more to the final weighted value. This puts emphasis on the older points, which again may be imprecise for the same reason. So, weighting factors that are greater than 1 do not help much in the healthcare case, either.

Boxcar averaging might be useful in some cases, but it is not very different from the subset sampling discussed previously; it just lumps together some of the data subsets. In short, time-weighting is fine for some other applications, but it is not likely to be helpful in healthcare because of the imprecise data being handled. If you wish to confirm or disprove this, Excel provides time-weighting functionality, and you can experiment.

SUMMING UP QUANTITATIVE ANALYSIS

Tracking data is fundamental to Six Sigma problem detection. The tracked data are average values and standard deviations using data from processes of interest. When the data sets are sparse, looking at confidence intervals is the better practice. When the data sets are rich, then straightforward application of spreadsheet functions AVERAGE(. . .) and STDEV.P(. . .) are quite good for your purposes.

Regression analysis can sometimes bring out the influence of parameters such as work-shift effects, winter-summer effects, or the like. All data and analysis are to be used cautiously because the starting data are likely to be imprecise. More data always help.

Problem Solving

Problems are solved by examining events, figuring out what went wrong, and deciding what might work better. Six Sigma provides a systematic management method for responding to events both to make sure that the event does not repeat itself and to be confident that long-term remedies are evaluated prudently before they are applied to the whole of the organization.

EVENTS

Causality

Chicago, October 8, 1871: Mrs. O'Leary's cow accidentally kicks over a kerosene lantern and sets fire to straw on the barn floor. The fire spreads, leaving 80,000 people homeless and 300,000 without drinking water. Twenty-six hundred acres of residential, commercial, and industrial real estate go up in smoke (Chicago Historical Society and the Trustees of Northwestern University 1996).

What caused this fire? The lantern? The dry straw? The dry weather? The cow? Historians have long since exonerated Mrs. O'Leary, but the official cause remains up for debate.

Aristotle said that every event has four causes (Magee 2015): a material cause, the formal cause, a proximate cause, and an efficient cause. The formal cause is not of much interest in practical matters, but the other three are. The efficient cause is the person who took the action that triggered the proximate cause, which in turn activated the material cause, all of which together caused the event to happen.

In Chicago on that fateful day, Mrs. O'Leary's abundant flammables were the material cause, the lantern was the proximate cause, and Mrs. O'Leary's cow was the efficient cause.

When looking at events, it is useful to start with Aristotle and sort out the material, proximate, and efficient causes, if only to have an immediate appreciation that every party involved will have two others to point at, each with some logic on his or her side. Without the other two causes, the event would not have happened at that time and place. It might have happened at another time and place, but if the focus is on exactly one event, every interested party can point at two others. The "flammables guy" can point at the lantern and the cow, the "lantern guy" can point at the flammables and the cow, and the cow . . . well, the cow cannot very well point and will probably wind up with the blame.

Chain of Events

Why was that lantern placed where the cow could knock it over? Who put the lantern there? Why was that person in the barn after dark? Why was a kerosene lantern being used instead of a safety lamp of some kind (remembering that this was 1871 and technology was somewhat quaint)? Why was the cow there, in the middle of Chicago? Who was in charge of the cow? Was the cow sufficiently constrained so as to preclude kicking over lanterns? Why was all that straw there? Why was it not wetted down to preclude ignition? Where was the nearest fire extinguisher? Who called the fire brigade? Where was the nearest fire station?

Walking through the chain of events is informative. Keeping in mind that three causes occur in chains of events is helpful, and trying to deal with everything in one chain often causes a jumble. Management needs to trace through the chains of events and take steps immediately to break those chains—or to break one of them at the very least—so that the same unhappy thing cannot happen again immediately. Not doing so would not be prudent management.

Yet this is not sufficient. The exact same chain of events will not likely happen again, but something similar may well happen, and it is important that steps be taken to anticipate such problems and find a more general solution.

THE THREE-PLANE MODEL

Some industries study events by considering them on three planes (exhibit 5.1):

1. Mechanisms
2. Conditions
3. Constraints

Exhibit 5.1: Three-Plane Model

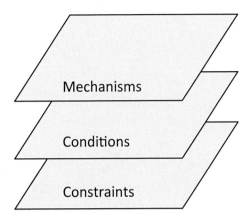

On the "mechanism" plane go the chains of events and mechanistic analyses, such as failure modes and effects.

On the "conditions" plane go the circumstances that applied to the development of the situation. For the Chicago fire, the circumstances were hot, dry weather; crowded construction; fire brigades sized to handle only two local fires a day; no fire-warning telegraph callboxes in residential areas; doubtful construction standards for residential areas; illumination by fire in lanterns and gas lamps; and horses and cows kept in residential areas.

On the "constraints" plane go the policies, regulations, laws, standards, and other administrative controls that bear on the circumstances. Again, in the case of the Chicago fire, these would include fire codes, zoning, brigade staffing rules, callbox placement, animal control regulations, and fire-watch staffing. The constraints plane is where management can control the conditions that govern the chain of events.

The city managers of Chicago might have considered the conditions and concluded that they could not do much about animal control because horses and cows were needed for transportation and milk production. They could not do much about construction standards because wooden construction was the only thing likely to be practicable in the Midwest. On the other hand, they could do something about construction density, perhaps carving out fire breaks by putting major road arteries every quarter of a mile or so to contain any future fire into one large square. They could add more fire stations. They could add more telegraph fire callboxes. They could require that a bucket of sand be kept in every barn. They could put up warning posters and enact laws against leaving lanterns unattended in barns. They could do several of these things, expecting more results from some than from others.

Sorting information out and putting it on these three conceptual planes (mechanisms, conditions, and constraints) takes time and effort. However, it is usually time and effort well-spent because it gives management a frame of reference to use when considering new policies.

DIGGING IN

An event has happened, and you want to know why. You want to know how to make sure, as best you can, that it does not happen again. It takes digging to find the facts; to find the chains of events; to find the circumstances; and to find the policies, rules, and regulations that were to be followed. Indeed, were they followed? If not, was it for a good reason?

When doing this digging, it is useful to find a comparable event that was "normal" so that distinctions can be found between the normal and the abnormal event. The first scientific principle is that effects flow from prior causes, so a change in outcome must flow from some change in the operation. Perhaps the change is due to normal fluctuations in operations; this matter will be taken up later in this book. At this point, we will attend to events that were sufficiently far out of the ordinary that they were called directly to the attention of management.

The management interest in digging into such events is to find something management can do to control future events. What policies need attention? What technology needs attention? What staffing or training need attention? What capital facilities need attention? What stop-gap measures should be implemented immediately to break the chain of events?

In doing the digging, some diagrammatic tools have been found to be helpful. These will be taken up shortly. Diagrams are helpful because, in most cases, the hard facts are only part of the story. People may well have seen different—even contradictory—things. People with an interest in the case may have different interests to protect or project. Any gaps in the story may be filled in differently by different people. Differences almost always are found between the stated policy on how things *should be* done and how they are *actually* done. These differences might be important, and they might not come to light if the investigation is not thorough.

People are naturally defensive if something untoward has happened on their watch. Defensive people are not very helpful at producing unbiased information. Getting the cooperation of these people, who are the very ones who probably know the most about what happened, is pretty important for getting to the bottom of problems.

Proceeding in a nonjudgmental way is important, and that is where diagrams come into play. The diagrams do not make any judgment, and they are one way of getting the cooperation of people who are not inclined to cooperate.

The best way to get such cooperation is to establish a track record of being non-judgmental, of treating people reasonably, and of not punishing the messenger. That takes time, and it takes a consistent approach across senior management, but it can be done. Indeed, one of the most important contributions executive management can make is to clarify the thinking on this matter for the middle management.

COMPARE

Start with the event itself and some comparable case that had the expected outcome. Figure out the chains of events. Get anecdotal input. Use group meetings and diagrams. Look for the input or operation that distinguishes the two cases. There must be at least one difference; several may be evident, but there will be at least one.

In some cases, a benchmark case is available that is thoroughly documented and that can serve as the reference case. When first starting out, benchmark cases may not be at hand, but as you apply the Six Sigma management method over time, benchmark cases will make themselves available naturally.

Dig deeper into each of the differences. Suspend judgment, if humanly possible, until all of the differences are understood. The rule of thumb is to dig until you think you have identified the source of the problem, then dig deeper, and then dig deeper again.

Compare

Study the event, and study a comparable event that had a normal outcome.

Benchmarks Help

As you apply Six Sigma, you will acquire benchmarks that will provide direct bases for comparison.

Although this can get out of hand, it is good to dig deep enough to be sure that nothing is hidden just below the present level of examination.

CATEGORIES OF DIFFICULTIES

We will now take a look at some likely categories of difficulties.

Worker Error

The first thing to do is to change the heading to something other than "Worker Error," because that starts the whole process with a witch-hunt ambiance. We will start again.

Design of Work

Did the event happen because of an error in carrying out a task? How is the work task designed? Does it conform to poka-yoke guidelines? Has the worker been trained and retrained? Does this task get done correctly on the day shift but not on the other shifts? Does this task get done correctly by some groups but not by other groups? What is the training or qualification policy that governs this task? How is the task actually done?

Experienced workers commonly ignore the official directions and perform tasks the way they think they should be done. Often, they are right; after all, they do the task all the time, and the efficiency expert who wrote the procedure is long gone. Sometimes, though, they are wrong, and it is necessary to find out what is really being done so that the matter can be sorted out.

Equipment Failure

Did the event happen because of an equipment failure? Equipment failure may not seem to be a management issue, but it is. Management needs to provide sufficient backup and fail-over equipment so that the combined system, with primary and backup equipment considered, is very robust. Therefore, the management interest is in knowing what backup equipment is on hand, how it is deployed, how people are trained to switch over to backups at the critical moment (which is when primary equipment always fails) without loss of function, and how the primary and backup equipment is maintained and certified for use.

If the backup equipment operates differently, the operators must be qualified to work on both the primary and backup equipment. If knobs are to be turned in the opposite direction on the backup equipment, trouble lurks.

Equipment breakdowns in this age of computer marvels are less frequent than they used to be, and this is a great thing. However, it also means that attention needs to be paid to making sure workers practice performing the switchover because they may never have done it in their normal course of work.

Hidden Equipment Malfunction

Did the event happen because of a hidden malfunction of the equipment? A serious question in the computer age is whether the equipment is working or not. Although a well-designed machine will provide a running display of what it is doing and keep track of its internal workings itself, with suitable reports to the operator, the machine is probably only checking itself on the inside. The machine probably cannot tell if its hoses are connected correctly or even if they are connected at all. The same is true for electrical leads and other connective devices.

External verification is important. This may be achieved with a separate instrument or by operator observation of signals distinct from those on the machine, such as patient manifestations or other indirect signs.

Although this is a system-level consideration and not a work-task consideration, system design can take advantage of poka-yoke, too. Is it easier for the operator to interpret the indirect signals correctly than not? Are mistakes (in this case, equipment malfunctions) immediately obvious? Does the operator have some means of correcting matters on the spot? Malfunction drills help, particularly drills that involve a whole team of people.

The ongoing computerization of healthcare raises such concerns. Computerization has its own chapter, later in this book.

Internal Surge in Demand

Was the event triggered by a surge in demand that for some reason was internal to the organization? Was this because of an emergency? A blunder in scheduling? A policy that helped one department by creating an overload in another? Was there, on the other hand, an unplanned shortfall in capacity because of personnel scheduling, fatigued staff, or an expected demand for personnel elsewhere?

External Surge in Demand

Was the event triggered by a surge in demand that was for some reason external to the organization? If so, the likelihood of something going wrong is increased. Although external events are by definition beyond the control of the organization, they raise the question of whether the organization has considered external events in its capacity planning in a reasonable way.

Forest fires occur in California every February. Forest fires usually mean injuries. But what severity of fire should a healthcare organization use for the basis of its planning? The fire that occurs once a century? Once every 50 years? The 1-year fire, or the 5-year fire?

If the facility is near a freeway where multicar accidents happen, is the organization prepared for the 50-year crash, the 10-year crash, or even the 1-year crash?

The same must be considered for building fires, factory explosions, earthquakes, floods, and other external events that can be predicted to happen at some time but not with any precision in the timing. What service level does management establish for such expected but unpredictable events? Does management have enough information in hand about the consequences of such events that a reasonable policy can be established?

Infrastructure

Did an infrastructure breakdown contribute to the event? Infrastructure is usually a combination of public services and internal backup services.

For example, water is purchased from the local water company, and in addition the facility has its own water tank with, for example, a four-hour inventory to take care of any upsets in the public supply. Is the sizing basis for the internal backup up to date? What is the public company's outage experience? Is some policy in place to cut down on water use while the internal tank is being employed? Does the facility engineer, management, or both know when water is being drawn from the internal tanks?

Take electricity as another example. Public electric supply is subject to outages. Most facilities of any size provide themselves with a local electric diesel generator that starts immediately when the public supply is interrupted. In addition, vital electrical loads have battery backup. Although the details of the diesel loading sequence and the maintenance of each battery system are a matter for the engineering staff, the management issue arises from the growth in electrical demand as more and more computerized devices are added. Is the demand following the established capacity plan? Is attention being paid by the electric company? Is the electric company providing two feeds to the facility so that one knocked-over pole someplace in its territory will not shut down electric service to the facility? Are the diesels up-to-date and ample in capacity? Is a rational sizing rule in place for each battery system? The same types of questions must be considered for communications systems and for any data networking and external computer services.

Services provided by trucks have the same characteristics and hardwired infrastructures. Consider the supplies of medicine, special gases, and other materials. What is the reliability of the external suppliers and trucking service providers? Is the inventory of each set by some reasonable rule based on robust service rather than on economic order quantities?

Unplanned Circumstances

Was the event caused by circumstances not considered in prior planning? For instance, if the patient care unit has three patients all named John J. Anderson, the normal type of patient nametag may not be of much use in keeping track if the nametag system design does not anticipate duplicate names. This situation would be even more serious if the nursery had three babies named John J. Anderson.

Unplanned Events

Was the event so unusual that it was simply beyond the planning bases that the organization has in place? Some maladies exist that few practitioners have seen, either because they are very near to eradication from the planet or because they only exist in some far-distant land. A traveler on safari in Kenya might acquire lion fever and bring it home, developing symptoms only on his or her return. Would any local doctor recognize lion fever? Is it reasonable that any local doctor should, or that the organization be prepared to deal with a lion fever case? Does the organization have a planning basis for responding to new demands for services that might be quite sudden in onset? Elective eye surgery for vision correction is a current example of this situation.

Willful Misconduct

And so we return to worker error. This time, we are discussing willful misconduct, dereliction of duty, substance abuse, sabotage, or a prank gone awry. This is not a matter of task design. This is a matter of an employee who wants to be an ex-employee.

Nothing weakens staff respect for management so quickly and thoroughly as a manifest ineptitude when it comes to dealing with problem employees, and this is deservedly so. Take care of the situation. Get rid of problem employees. Get rid of problem managers, too.

GENERALIZING THE SOLUTION

After management is confident that it has identified the chain of events and the causes of the event, it needs to be sure that a solution is provided that definitively covers the particular event and, in addition, covers the general class of events exemplified by the particular case. Finding that general solution usually falls to management because it almost always involves a change in policy, a change in technology, or a change in capital facilities.

Solutions

Seek a particular solution and seek a general solution. The general solution usually requires management action.

A change in technology has the advantage that it can be given a trial run, and any concomitant issues can be seen and addressed. Changes in policy are hard to implement on a trial-run basis; the change either is the new policy or it is not the new policy. It is also hard to make changes in a capital facility on a trial basis. Once the concrete is poured, it is a little late to discover and fix any awkward features of a new building. One possibility is to do the trial somewhere else. Find a similar organization that has already established the new policy or built a comparable facility. Visit it, scrutinize it, and dig out the anecdotes as well as the facts and figures.

CAUTION

No solution is ever guaranteed. Every change in an organization, whether it is a policy change, a technology change, or a capital facility change, needs to be made with a great deal of care and caution. Managing change is a key facet of Six Sigma, and it is covered later in this book.

POSITIVE APPLICATIONS

Not all events are bad; some are surprisingly good. The same management approach that gets you to an understanding of an untoward event and its causes will work just as well with a positive event. Applying this approach systematically to positive events is a sound way to improve overall performance. This may even be considered the management of serendipity.

Most scientific discoveries are made this way—not by accident exactly but by seizing on fortunate happenings. Being observant is the second requisite; being curious is the third. Being ready to follow up and dig in to understand what is causing the favorable result is the fourth benefit.

Benefit from Creativity

1. Encourage
2. Observe
3. Be curious
4. Understand
5. Capitalize

Any organization may have employees who are creative in their work. They find easier ways to do things to save themselves some time and effort. This is not cutting corners. It is creativity.

Management has the responsibility of encouraging responsible creativity at all levels for the simple reason that management does not have the energy or the opportunity to do all the creative work itself. Help from all ranks should be appreciated.

When the Six Sigma management system is mature in an organization, all key processes are tracked. From the tracking charts, it is just as easy to see a favorable event as an unfavorable event. The unfavorable events have their own way of demanding attention. Management is responsible for paying attention to the favorable events, too.

DIAGRAMMATIC TOOLS

Failure Modes and Effects Analysis

The idea of the failure modes and effects analysis is to link events, usually without much consideration of the likelihood of any particular event or combination of events. More elaborate forms include probabilistic weighting, but that is beyond what is likely to be needed for management purposes in dealing with some untoward event, either real or hypothetical.

The failure modes and effects analysis can be performed by looking from the effects back to the causes or from the causes forward to their effects. For example, consider this effect: A wheel comes off the mail cart. What can cause this? The wheel itself could break, the cart leg could break, the axle could break, the cotter pin could come out of the axle, or the shank of the leg down where the axle goes through it could get bent so that the axle could pop out. We could then go further back to ask, What would cause the axle to break? Well, the answer may be poor lubrication, material defect, destructive handling during assembly, abrasion against the strut, chemical attack by the disinfectant used to wash the cart, and so on. Similar lists could be developed for each of the other potential causes of the wheel coming off.

Alternatively, we could go in the other direction and ask, what happens if the wheel comes off? Well, the cart might tip, mail could be dumped on the floor, mail would be held up, some mail might get lost, the aisle could be blocked by the wreckage, the cart user might be injured by the spill, another cart going by might be tipped in turn, the floor might get gouged, or a passerby might get a pocketful of mail.

These types of diagrams, such as in exhibit 5.2, are commonly drawn out in a tree. Before computers came along, they were drawn on the back of wallpaper rolls. They can be done by hand on a blackboard if the exercise is restricted to likely events and significant consequences.

It may be helpful to ask the following:

1. How is this process supposed to work?
2. Where are the obvious weak spots at which something might fail?
3. If failure transpires, what are the consequences?
4. If such consequences are significant, can some change be proposed to mitigate those particular consequences?

Exhibit 5.2: Failure Modes and Effects Example

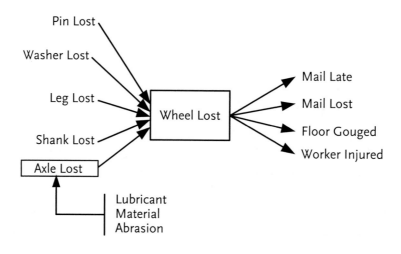

If some change is proposed, restart the process and think again through weak spots, failure modes, and consequences.

Predicting every eventuality is impossible. Reasonable effort should be put into thinking the situation through, looking for potential problems, and thinking about failure modes and effects, but those will never replace some actual experience (most likely experience acquired in a trial run).

NASA has lost, sad to say, a small number of astronauts in the past 40 years; each was lost in an accident. In no case had that accident been foreseen in a prior failure modes and effects analysis, even though NASA had committed to such analyses to an exhaustive degree precisely in an effort to preclude the loss of astronauts. NASA's failure modes and effects analysis work, with an unlimited budget, was not and could not have been 100 percent complete. The proof of this is that the analysis was done, designs were improved to preclude loss, and a few astronauts were lost anyway. The point is this: Failure modes and effects analyses are tools to be used, but they are not the totality of the problem-solving effort.

Even with these limitations, failure modes and effects analysis will focus attention on ripple effects and provide an organized means to identify and preclude a large portion of the ripples beforehand. A complementary method known as potential problem analysis will be discussed later.

Fishbone Analysis

The existing system got the way it is for various good reasons over the life of the organization. Certainly, these reasons seemed pretty solid at the time the existing management policy was put in place. Changing things now will work best if the decision-making process includes an understanding of how things got the way they are.

Informing the affected parties is a pretty good policy. Getting input from these parties is also a pretty good policy. Getting input from various ranks in the organization is, again, a pretty good policy. These policies are to be weighed against the likelihood of reinventing the present system or running out of time to do anything.

A useful tool to apply at the gathering-views stage is the fishbone diagram, which is also called an *Ishikawa diagram*. This tool is useful in gathering and organizing input without applying any judgment to the value of the input, at least not while the diagram is being made. In other words, this tool is useful in defusing meetings by getting everybody's input onto one chart. Part of the input is very likely to be a discussion of why the present system is the way it is. This is informative for the rest of the group, and it may give rise to better suggestions for improvement.

A suitable candidate for change is one that deals with one or more of the issues on the fishbone diagram. To put it another way, unless the change candidate deals with one or more of the issues on the fishbone diagram, the change is not going to make any difference.

The fishbone diagram is not a chain of events, and it does not distinguish very well among mechanisms, conditions, and constraints. This is okay; it is still a good place to start. The information can be sorted out later into the three-plane model.

Exhibit 5.3 shows an example of a fishbone diagram that looks at the various possible causes of delay in getting a patient transferred by cart from one patient care unit to another.

Exhibit 5.3: Example of a Fishbone Diagram

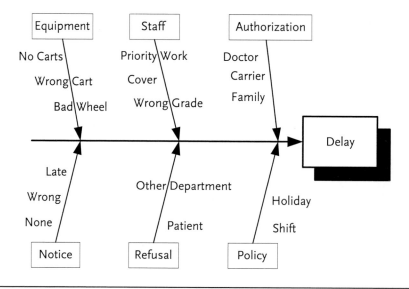

The fishbone diagram itself does not prioritize anything or give more weight to one item than to another. The point, at this stage of the analysis, is to be inclusive.

MANAGEMENT ACTION

If it is immediately obvious that a new policy will solve the problem forevermore, management should institute that policy. This, unfortunately, is almost never the case. Sorting out issues, considering alternatives, thinking things through, and testing the best candidates for new policies takes time and effort. Therefore, management needs to proceed in a step-by-step fashion:

1. Institute a stop-gap measure to break the chain(s) of events.
2. Authorize a study group to consider the chain(s) of events, the circumstances, and the policies now in force and to propose new policies.
3. Expect the study group to create fishbone diagrams and perform other cause-and-effect fact gathering and information gathering.
4. Expect the study group to identify the chain(s) of events.
5. Expect the study group to apply the three-plane model.
6. Expect the study group to recommend new constraints in the form of new management policies or actions.
7. Authorize a trial of the proposed new policies.
8. Evaluate the trial.
9. Apply the new policy in a general way if the trial is successful.
10. Monitor results on a long-term basis to be confident that circumstances have not changed in some adverse way over time.

The "policy change" is quite often a technology change, which is to say that the new policy is to use technology X rather than the prior technology Y. Such decisions may require substantial funding and may take time to implement. Meanwhile, the stop-gap measures must be kept in place.

Any policy or technology change needs to be tested carefully in a trial before it is applied universally. How to manage that trial will be discussed later in this book.

JOINT COMMISSION SENTINEL EVENTS

The Joint Commission (2016a) mandates specific actions for sentinel events. A Joint Commission sentinel event, then, is a manifestation of a problem that needs to be solved. The Six Sigma method for problem solving conforms to The Joint Commission requirements for analyzing and preventing the recurrence of sentinel events. This method is not restricted to such serious matters as sentinel events; the same systematic method can be applied to both great matters and small matters. Indeed, having some experience with small and medium-sized matters is good preparation for dealing with a life-threatening event.

ROOT CAUSES

The Joint Commission has a specific definition of root causes that it wishes to see applied in analyses done for sentinel events. The general notion is that pulling out the cause at its root solves the problem for good. However, this presupposes that the root cause can be found, that something can be done about it, and that that something is within the control of the organization's management. None of these is necessarily true.

A three-plane analysis is useful for seeking root causes. Sometimes the root cause is merely a breakdown in the mechanism, which is cured by replacing or upgrading the mechanism. More often, the root cause is found on the conditions plane, and dealing with the root cause—pulling the root out—requires some management action toward change, and this will show up on the constraints plane.

Here are a few examples:

Condition	Constraint
Patients move around of their own volition, including wandering off the premises.	Change policy to restrict movement past the property line, and reinforce it with alarm technology.
Visitors carry newborn babies out of the maternity rooms.	Change policy to restrict the movement of babies by visitors to same room.
Employees carry laptop computers home to do extra work. Some computers get lost.	Change policy to require any such employees to carry insurance against such loss.

Breaking a chain of events is different from pulling out a root cause. Take the example cited in the conditions/constraints table above dealing with employees who take computers home to do additional work. There is a way to break the chain of events: Forbid employees from taking computers home. However, if the employee cannot take the computer home, he or she is not going to do that report, special assignment, or self-help study, and the organization surely wants to encourage all of those things. Perhaps requiring the employee to carry insurance against loss of the organization's computers is a better solution, even if the organization gives the employee money to cover the additional insurance cost. Perhaps better solutions or different constraints could address the condition, protect the organization's interests, and avoid discouraging employees from doing extra work outside the office.

The mechanisms leading to a specific event are themselves quite specific—so specific, in fact, that breaking the chain of events probably only precludes that specific event from happening again. Other events of the same class may still happen because their mechanics are slightly different. To find a more general solution (to pull the root cause), look at the conditions and constraints that are general, not specific, and apply the three-plane model discussed earlier.

It is to be noted that root cause analysis is often criticized as being too mechanical and very likely missing important human factors (Cassin and Barach 2012). After doing a root cause analysis, it is prudent to stand back, ask what human and organizational factors may have colored various inputs, and then apply any conclusions cautiously.

Communications and Teams

Communications need to take account of inadvertent error. To do so, apply the now-familiar three rules:

1. Design the communication so that success is more likely than failure.

2. Let the sender determine if the communication succeeded or failed.

3. Let the sender make a correction on the spot.

DESIGN FOR SUCCESS

Eschew pronouns. Pronouns invite ambiguity. Pronouns are never necessary. There are whole books, including this one, that contain very few pronouns.

Disambiguate. Be aware of medical terms that sound a great deal like each other, and take care to distinguish one from another.

Use the phonetic alphabet. Alpha, Bravo, Charlie, Delta, Echo, Foxtrot, Golf, Hotel, India, Juliette, Kilo, Lima, Mike, November, Oscar, Papa, Quebec, Romeo, Sierra, Tango, Uniform, Victor, Whiskey, X-ray, Yankee, Zulu. One, Too, T'ree, Fow-er, Fife, Six, Sev-en, Eight, Nin-er, Zee-ro. These words are immediately understood by the receiving party, and none sounds like another. This is particularly important with numbers, because the English words for numbers are not very distinct as conventionally pronounced. Say the numbers one at a time because, for example, *seventeen* and *seventy* are easily confused, while *one sev-en* and *sev-en zee-ro* are easily distinguished.

REPLY

The action moves to the receiving party, but the responsibility rests with the sender. The sender must require that the receiving party respond before taking any action that impinges on the patient.

The receiving party needs to communicate back to the sender that the message has been received and comprehended. "Yes, ma'am" does the first but not the second. Silence does neither.

The same applies for written as well as verbal communications.

If there is no reply, or if the reply is not sufficient, then the sender has no basis on which to decide if the communication was a success or a failure. The responsibility resides with the sender, so the sender must insist.

CORRECTION

If the sender determines that a correction is required, the communications task needs to start again. Furthermore, the process needs to have been designed to allow time for a corrective message or for mitigation after the fact. Allowing a little time seems to be the better course.

TEAMS

There are one-party communications, usually notes written to self. Most healthcare work, though, is done by several people assembled in teams, so error-resistant communication is key.

Surgical Teams

Talk about stress!

The stress is unavoidable, so the question is, can outcomes be improved by improving communications?

Dr. Paul Barach, an important figure in patient safety and an anesthesiologist by specialization, focuses on the human factors of pediatric cardiac surgery.

Dr. Atul Gawande (2009), surgeon, has written extensively on his own journey to find the best way to manage his surgical team in the interest of the patient. Dr. Gawande does not have a standing team to work with but rather draws nurses and anesthesiologists from pools so that each surgery has a new team. To ensure a smooth procedure, Dr. Gawande moves systematically through the following process.

Before starting, Dr. Gawande reviews the patient's history out loud. Each person around the table is asked in turn to remark on any particular considerations, such as allergy to anesthetics. Dr. Gawande states out loud what he will do in the first surgical step and reads through a short checklist. He then executes the first surgical step, stops, invites comments, goes through a new checklist. And so on.

While all surgeons tell everyone to speak up and some even mean it, Dr. Gawande actually has everybody talking. That's a big difference, whether or not the team members are used to each other.

Ad Hoc Teams

Code or Code Blue events in hospitals trigger a call for all hands to rush to the bed of a patient undergoing cardiac arrest. The first one to get there starts doing something; there is no waiting for the whole team to assemble or to go through a preflight rehearsal. For the first several minutes, no one is in charge and yet the team is doing lifesaving work.

The University of Pittsburgh's Peter M. Winter Institute for Simulation, Education, and Research—WISER for short—has developed training programs for such personnel, shown in exhibit 6.1 and summarized as follows (DeVita et al. 2004):

Exhibit 6.1: Diagram of Code Events Stations

Code Event Stations

- The positions around the bed are assigned a number.
- Each position is assigned specific tasks.
- Each person arriving takes up an open position for which that person is qualified.
- No one changes position, even if a more-qualified person comes in.
- Drills help.

Relay Teams

Relay team members cooperate only at the moment of handoff, passing the baton.

Passing the baton looks like a simple thing, yet even so there are ways of doing things. In a short race, the runner with the baton is responsible for slapping the baton firmly into the hand of the next runner, whose head is turned the other way. In a longer race, the fresh runner looks back and is responsible for grasping the baton from the flagging runner.

In healthcare, the patient is handed over several times. An emergency patient is handed from the Emergency Department to a Medical-Surgical Department, then perhaps to X-Ray and Surgery, perhaps to the Intensive Care Unit (ICU), then to another Medical-Surgical Department, to Rehab, before step-down care and home care, and perhaps more. While in the hospital, the patient will have the attention of a case worker who makes sure each step is taken, and taken in a timely manner. Over the entire sequence, there is no single person who is directing the actions. The patient's primary care physician gets reports, but the primary care physician is pretty far away from the action.

So, as in a relay race, each leg is autonomous, and each handoff is vital to success.

Solo Relay

Solo relay? Self-relay? The point is that communications between people are fallible and always introduce some chance of things going awry. One way to avoid this is to reduce the number of responsible parties, letting one person take on consecutive tasks. The person needs to be qualified for each task, of course.

Task-by-task specialization, and therefore relaying, is efficient and ensures the greatest proficiency at each step. That's good. Having one person perform two consecutive tasks is likely to be less efficient when measured task by task.

In the bigger picture, however, with credit for the elimination of at least one relay handover, maybe the overall error count will go down.

SURGERY ICU TO MEDICAL-SURGICAL TRANSFER

Standards require that the receiving nurse be allowed to ask questions of the ICU nurse. This is not quite up to Six Sigma standards because the receiving nurse is made responsible for the communication. If questions are to be asked, it would be better if the ICU nurse asks the questions, after conveying the information, so that the ICU nurse, as the responsible party, is confident that the receiving nurse understood everything.

NURSING-SHIFT CHANGE

When the shift changes, responsibility for the patient passes from one nurse to another. It is good practice for both nurses to go the patient's room and take up positions on two sides of the bed. Nurse A reviews matters for Nurse B. Both nurses examine IV insertion points and the like. The patient can speak up to the benefit of both nurses.

HOSPITAL DISCHARGE

The literature is replete with data saying that patients don't remember doctors' instructions and generally misunderstand whatever instructions they do remember (Lieber 2015). Hospitals work hard to do better in this area. For example, the discharge nurse will take the time to instruct the patient on any follow-up care and then have the patient "teach it back." This closes the loop and gives the nurse the opportunity to verify that the patient understood what is to be done and to correct misunderstandings as necessary. Discharge does not occur until the instructions are understood and are confirmed to be understood. This conforms to the three Six Sigma rules, because the teach-it-back step allows the nurse to distinguish success from failure and to fix problems on the spot.

COMPUTER-TO-COMPUTER COMMUNICATIONS

Computer-to-computer communications are very carefully designed and tested because computers don't have any sense. Six Sigma computer-to-computer communications require the following:

- Computer-to-computer messages are specific.
- A message that does not conform to a known list of proper messages is rejected and reported back to sender.
- Messages that contain noise are rejected and reported back to sender.
- Successful messages are acknowledged back to sender.
- The sending computer will raise an exception if no feedback, positive or negative, is received in a timely manner.

In this last point, the sending computer is taking responsibility insofar as a computer can take responsibility in any meaningful way. At least the sending computer raises an exception and bumps the exception report up to the eventual attention of a human being. Timeliness and prioritization—both of which are computer system design issues not peculiar to messaging—then come into question.

DOCTOR'S ORDERS

Consider a doctor's orders for hospital care:

- Once the order is written, the action moves to the responsible nurse.
- The nurse will observe that the order is within a customary range of orders for the stated diagnosis.
- The nurse will check drug names and dosages against customary practices for the stated diagnosis and patient weight.
- The nurse will call the doctor before taking action if the nurse finds anything amiss or exceptional.
- The nurse *will not* call the doctor before taking action if the nurse finds the order to be ordinary.

This conforms only in part to Six Sigma task-design rules. The doctor does not know if the order was received and understood prior to the nurse's taking actions that might impinge upon the patient, and there is no possibility that the doctor can correct an inadvertent error before actions impinge upon the patient.

While this has been accepted practice for more than a hundred years, in this day of instantaneous messaging, it would seem to be possible to close the communications loop prior to actions being taken so that the responsibility resides with the doctor and inadvertent error can be dealt with at the right point in the process. See "Message Overload and the Time Basis for Computer-to-Person Communications" in chapter 8.

ELECTRONIC PATIENT RECORD NARRATIVE

Doctors and nurses are getting used to entering data into electronic records, checking boxes, typing in numbers, and writing or dictating a narrative. Concern has been expressed that both doctors and nurses are devoting less attention to filling in the narrative portion than in the past. As the point of the narrative is to record that which the box-checking doesn't convey, either this needs attention or the narrative concept should be abandoned.

The narrative does not conform to any of the three Six Sigma rules for task design. There are no standards for content of the narrative. The receiving party is not identified. There is no feedback path. The narrator cannot know if the narrative content was received and understood; therefore, corrections cannot be made in a timely manner.

The role of the narrative in this age of electronic records needs further consideration.

Workflow

Find the bottleneck, because the bottleneck determines the output of the entire system. Manage upstream and downstream to maximize bottleneck performance. And don't forget interruptions!

THE LEAN CONCEPT

Making the best use of capital investment and labor has been a management goal, always. In recent years, the various ways of getting to that best use have been captured under the rubric "Lean," which used to be "Lean Manufacturing." The principles are applied far beyond manufacturing, so dropping the earlier rubric is in order.

The original idea was to reduce work-in-process inventory without reducing production. That's a worthy goal—to reduce the number of dollars tied up in inventory. However, work-in-process inventory reduction is not a bell-ringer in healthcare; indeed, there are plenty of places where having a superfluity of inventory is a really good idea. Still, the fundamental point, that the flow of work can be analyzed and improved, abides. The approach of this book is to divide the overall process up by identifying the production bottleneck and then identifying what's upstream of the bottleneck and what's downstream of the bottleneck. There is always exactly one bottleneck (Smith, Barry, and Brubaker 2007). Understanding that bottleneck is the key to managing the operation.

Consider a patient care process. The measure of success is the rate at which treatments are successfully completed; what counts is the rate at which work flows through the organization. One item of work is one patient, and getting the patient to "flow" through the treatment facility in the minimum amount of time is the best use of the facility. Poor workflow leads to higher census and higher treatment costs for the same number of successful treatments. The organization and the facility have all kinds of constraints on capacity, and those constraints need to be understood so that the workflow can be managed in the best way.

THE BOTTLENECK

Consider the office of a family dentist, a sole practitioner with an established practice. Let us take a look at the workflow in the dentist's office. First of all, there is a bottleneck, which can be identified as the dentist herself. Suppose our dentist takes 20 minutes off in the middle of the afternoon; that represents 20 minutes of time with no production. Will patients wait an extra 20 minutes so that our dentist can make up the lost production by extending her workday 20 minutes? Maybe, but a patient might walk out, and more than one patient might start shopping for a more committed dentist. Can the dentist make up for the lost production by working faster on the next three patients? Maybe, but hurrying might trigger an error that would then take even more time to correct, thereby delaying production all the more and putting the patient in question on the list of those shopping for a new dentist. In short, any productive time lost at the bottleneck is production lost forever.

Furthermore, any productive time lost at the bottleneck *for any reason* is production lost forever. If the patient is late, if the patient's records are not in order, if the dentist's drills are not cleaned and ready, if the Novocain supply runs out, if the hand tools are not out of the sterilizer, if the bib supply runs out, if any of a million little things goes wrong, productive time is lost forever. Knowing this, the dentist makes an effort to make sure that everything is ready and to double-check her system before each patient is put in the chair. Meanwhile, pains are taken to make sure the patient arrives and that payment is ensured by checking the insurance authorization before the patient gets in the chair.

So, with the patient present and qualified and with the system double-checked, the bottleneck work gets under way. This is the most productive the dentist can make her office. The dentist also makes sure that as little dead time as possible transpires between patients. Cleaning up after one patient and getting ready for the next is nonproductive time. Our dentist may invest in a second room and chair so that the setup time for each successive patient is near zero; this maximizes productive time at the bottleneck.

Suppose the dentist's son graduates from dental school and joins the practice. Suddenly there is a twofold expansion of the bottleneck; suddenly there is spare capacity; suddenly the practice is scrambling to expand the clientele population and thinking up new services to offer to soak up that excess capacity. Over time, this growth in clientele should fill up the new, expanded bottleneck.

Let us suppose, however, that no way is found to get the clientele population up to twice the former level. What should the dentists do? They should reduce capacity because having idle capacity is pointless. The dentist's son might go back to school part-time to study laser bonding to expand the service offerings. The dentist herself might take one day off a week to contribute her time to a charity clinic or to write the definitive book on dental practice.

Our dentists probably considered the market pretty carefully before they decided to double the capacity of their little organization, so they were likely able to fill the new capacity pretty quickly. Their business is simple to analyze, and because they run the business themselves, they surely thought things through before making the change.

Upstream

You know how dentists deal with things upstream of the bottleneck (the bottleneck being themselves). Patients are booked to arrive several minutes before the dentist actually plans to see them so that any minor lateness on the part of the patient does not trigger a loss of production in the bottleneck. The reception clerk checks records and insurance formalities before the patient gets called to the chair.

Suppose the standard dental treatment time is 20 minutes and the standard reception processing time is 5 minutes. The reception clerk can process four patients in the time it takes the dentist to do one. Should the reception clerk then work ahead, processing as many patients as he or she can to be as productive as possible? No! The reception clerk should be *idle* 15 minutes out of every 20. Getting extra patients in and processed only means that patients will be waiting longer to see the dentist, fuming all the while and contemplating what to tell the neighbors about the high-handedness of this dentist. Keeping the reception clerk busy is not a goal of the organization.

The reception clerk may be given other, low-priority duties to soak up idle time, but the standing orders to the reception clerk are to have the next patient processed before the dentist is ready for that patient and with a few minutes' slack. Attention is paid to the bottleneck because the bottleneck is the limit on production.

Downstream

The discharge clerk should process the outgoing patient promptly, so that outgoing patients do not get stacked up at the discharge desk, and sympathetically, so that the patients do not contemplate shopping for a different dentist.

Suppose the standard discharge-processing time is 5 minutes, and suppose our dentists' treatment time is again 20 minutes. The discharge clerk should be idle 15 minutes out of every 20. The discharge clerk should certainly not make patients sit around and wait until a sufficient batch of them is available to make the discharge clerk's work as productive as possible.

The discharge clerk may be given other, low-priority duties, such as making sure the magazines on the rack are sufficiently out of date so that patients are not tempted to sit down in the waiting room to finish that article, thereby clogging up the space. The standing orders to the discharge clerk are always to get that outgoing patient moved promptly, dropping other work to attend to the outgoing patient. The productivity of the discharge clerk is not important because the bottleneck is the limit on production, not the discharge clerk.

Kanban

Dentists always knew what Japanese factory managers discovered for themselves and called Kanban. Kanban is the anglicized version of the Japanese word for "punch card." The work-authorization form was a punch-card, and the name for the card came to be the name for the production strategy.

The Japanese decided that the right way to run a factory is to keep the work flowing continuously through the factory bottleneck and to keep those workers upstream of the bottleneck *idle* until they are authorized to produce work to flow into the bottleneck. Kanban works for factories just as it works for dentists' offices.

Goldratt's Model

Goldratt and Cox (1984) have elaborated Kanban into a general theory of production. The essence of the Goldratt theory is as follows:

1. The production of the bottleneck is the production of the organization.
2. Production upstream of the bottleneck should be on-demand and idle until demand arises.

3. Production downstream of the bottleneck should be idle until work comes to it from the bottleneck.

Is this not a simple theory? Does not every dentist already know this? Yet this theory is profound. Every organization has a bottleneck. Every organization has activities upstream of the bottleneck. Every organization has activities downstream of the bottleneck. To be specific, every healthcare service has a bottleneck, has activities upstream of the bottleneck, and has activities downstream of the bottleneck. Recognizing this truism is important because the management interest in each of the three phases is distinct.

WHY IS THERE A BOTTLENECK?

A bottleneck exists because the cost of expanding the bottleneck is so great as to be prohibitive. In financial terms, the cost to expand the bottleneck is so great that a negative financial impact continues throughout the financial planning period. This cost might be the cost of the extra dentist in our case above, the cost of building an expansion of the pediatric care unit, or the cost of another magnetic resonance imaging (MRI) machine. The limit might be the shortage of skilled personnel such as heart surgeons or specialized nurses.

In healthcare, bottlenecks may be created by regulation, such as a limit on the number of beds set by a regional commission. Bottlenecks may be imposed by the size of the physical facilities. There is always *one* bottleneck.

What happens if so many dentists offer services in a town that there are not enough patients to go around and no prospect of much growth in demand? Is that not the absence of a bottleneck? Yes, and the right response is to reduce capacity until a bottleneck occurs again. Drive the weakest practices out, buy up some others, and get the capacity down. If this does not happen, the aggregate economics are ruinous. In businesses with any prospect of survival, there is always a bottleneck.

Bottlenecks

- Every service has a true bottleneck resulting from physical capacity limits or regulations.
- If work is piling up elsewhere, there is an error in workflow management.
- Do not overcommit the bottleneck; save something as surge capacity.
- Do not worry about capacity in non-bottleneck locations because these locations can always catch up.

MANAGEMENT AT THE BOTTLENECK

Because any delay that affects the bottleneck affects the organization as a whole in direct measure, the operational focus is on making sure the bottleneck equipment is in order, all supplies are on hand, the staff are trained up to high standards, the patient is double-checked, and all patient records are double-checked. Any lost production at the bottleneck cannot be recovered, so the focus has to be on making sure that no production is lost at the bottleneck.

Any setup time at the bottleneck, even such mundane things as making up a bed, requires management attention to make sure that it is done correctly and promptly, because setup time is a direct detractor to the capacity of the bottleneck and therefore a direct detractor to the capacity of the entire system.

Both work and management at the bottleneck are intense. On the other hand, the bottleneck is easy to manage because the employees can see exactly how important their work is, there is plenty of work to do, and management is paying attention. Budgets for upkeep and upgrade are easily justified.

Management Upstream of the Bottleneck

The focus upstream of the bottleneck is on making sure the patient is ready to go to the bottleneck when the bottleneck is ready for the patient. Working ahead is not productive and is likely to annoy the patient by creating long waits in queue.

Workers upstream are idle much of the time. They need to be idle so that they can jump into action when triggered by notice from the bottleneck.

Having idle workers is anathema to the cost accounting department. Workers themselves do not like to be idle, especially skilled workers. And yet that is the optimum production strategy: capacity on-call (or, to say it another way, idleness until called) upstream of the bottleneck. This practice is accepted for firefighters (one wonders how cost accounting works for a fire brigade . . .), and it should be accepted for any activity that jumps into action when the call comes.

While upstream of the bottleneck, firefighters play checkers and wash the truck. Upstream healthcare workers can take up lower-priority work when idle from their main duties, or they can play checkers, as long as they stay at the ready for their principal duties when the call comes. Although the patient is the most important workflow item, the same logic applies to any department that feeds into the bottleneck department, including supplies, pharmacy, records, accounts, and so on.

Investments to increase capacity upstream are suspect, given that excess capacity already exists. Projects that would reduce capacity upstream are possible if capital assets are freed up and the projects are designed so that no new bottleneck is created.

Management Downstream of the Bottleneck

Downstream of the bottleneck, there is nothing to do until the work presents itself. Downstream there is excess capacity, so any minor loss of production is not a loss of production by the organization. A complete breakdown downstream will eventually stall the bottleneck and become a limit on the production of the organization.

Workers and equipment will be idle between episodes of work. Workers can be given low-priority work to fill the idle minutes, but the standing order has to be to jump-to when the work arrives. This is easy to manage, although most professional employees do not welcome idleness.

Investments to increase capacity downstream are suspect, given that excess capacity already exists. Projects that would reduce capacity downstream are possible if capital assets are freed up and the projects are designed so that no new bottleneck is created.

Bottleneck Placement

By and large, the nature of each organization dictates where the bottleneck will be. The extent to which management can control the placement of the bottleneck may indicate how easily it can see where the best place would be. The best place for the bottleneck is *not* at the end of the process. Everyone who shops at a grocery store is infuriated by the grocery store bottleneck: the checkout counters.

The right place to have a bottleneck is at the first step in the process. Some big-name theme parks restrict the number of patrons allowed into the park at one time so that the patrons will not have to wait interminably in queue to ride the popular rides. They put the bottleneck at the first step of their service process; that is the best place to have it.

Even though the ideal place for the bottleneck is recognized, most organizations find that their bottleneck is in the middle just by the nature of the business, and management can do nothing about it. The ideal is not attainable.

BOTTLENECKS AND BARRIERS

A major hospital expanded its MRI capacity by buying new machines. Patient throughput stayed the same. Upon inspection, it became obvious that the dressing rooms were now too small. Did the bottleneck move? No, because the dressing rooms were expanded with a minor investment of time and money. The dressing rooms were a barrier but not a bottleneck. A barrier can be expanded, but a bottleneck cannot be. So, when a barrier crops up, knock the barrier down.

MANAGING THE WORKFLOW

Three management regimes apply to the three segments of the workflow (bottleneck, upstream, and downstream). Because an organization's production rests on its production at the bottleneck, workflow management must start from the bottleneck and work in both directions, following these steps:

1. *Identify the bottleneck.* Apply maximum-net-production management rules to the bottleneck activity. Work to reduce nonproductive bottleneck time, such as machine setup time or room changeover time. Have workers on the bench to pinch-hit for absent productive personnel. Work on preventive maintenance, skill training, and retention. Analyze every detail, and look to improve yield. Apply poka-yoke to every task because any error in the bottleneck will take time to fix and will reduce productive capacity.
2. *Identify upstream work.* Apply idle-until-called-on management rules for upstream activity. Reduce variability to reduce the risk of being late to the bottleneck. Think poka-yoke. Check thoroughly for errors and correct them on the spot because errors propagating into the bottleneck are not desired.
3. *Identify downstream work.* Apply idle-until-work-arrives management rules for downstream activity. Reduce variability to reduce risk of backing workflow up into the bottleneck. Think poka-yoke. Check thoroughly for errors and correct them on the spot.

Or, one can consider the negative expression of these rules:

1. Do not lose production at the bottleneck for want of preparation or for want of double-checking the equipment, the staff, and the patient prior to doing the bottleneck work. Do not make mistakes in the bottleneck that will require rework in the bottleneck and a loss of production.
2. Do not confuse busyness with production upstream, thereby risking a loss of work for the bottleneck by failing to have the upstream staff or facilities ready to respond to the call. Do not make mistakes upstream that will propagate into the bottleneck.
3. Do not confuse busyness with production downstream, which may cause queuing up of patients, even to the extreme of backing up into the

bottleneck. Do not invite mistakes downstream that will back work up into the bottleneck or send rework back to the bottleneck.

SURGE CAPACITY

Honda is a well-managed Japanese car manufacturer. The Honda practice is to commit no more than 80 percent of a factory's capacity so that, if something goes wrong at the factory bottleneck, surge capacity is available to catch up to commitments. The financial argument against this policy is obvious because it means that 20 percent of the factory's capacity is not used most of the time, with a concomitant low return on assets.

This is an interesting balancing of interests. To keep customers happy, hold back some surge capacity so that the organization can catch up quickly to commitments. To keep accountants happy, hold nothing back. Honda thinks customers are more important than accountants. What do you think? Twenty percent may be too much surge capacity for most organizations, but zero is probably too little. Management should consider the Honda management model and make a conscious policy decision. Dentists might make a policy of not booking a half-hour in the middle of the afternoon to provide for some surge capacity.

THE KINDS OF WAITS

Workflow involves the transfer of patients or material from one work center to another. In healthcare, this is unlikely to be done by assembly line, so the workflow rate is not going to be uniform. Because the flow is not uniform, some time will be spent waiting. It is instructive to consider the different types of waiting that apply.

Removing all waits is not possible, but knowing what types of waits exist, which ones are there on purpose, and which ones are not, is a good idea. Waiting consumes resources because waiting extends the treatment time.

Queuing

Queuing is waiting for service. Queuing is appropriate and even necessary at the bottleneck because it is important to the organization that the bottleneck never run out of work.

The length of the queue at the bottleneck can be set in a design rule such as, "a queue of sufficient length such that the likelihood that the bottleneck will run out of work is less than 1 percent on any day."

This turns on two things: the predictability of the workload in the bottleneck and the predictability of the time required to move the next patient to the bottleneck. Both are amenable to study and quantification.

Pending

Pending is waiting for administrative release. Because this is not exactly the same as waiting for physical work to be completed, pending waits are largely under administrative control.

Consider the administrative step of getting the attending physician to discharge a patient. Some physical or mental work is required of the physician to review the case and sign the release. The administrative part is finding the physician, presenting the file, and waiting for the discharge order to be signed. This can be improved by providing roller skates to the file messenger, electronic mail to the physician, or other suitable means.

Other administrative tasks may be pending, such as social service reports, family authorizations, rehabilitation facility acceptance, credit approvals, and so on. Each needs to be addressed in a distinct way because any improvement will not likely apply across the board when dealing with such a varied population.

Batching

Batching is the intentional grouping of patients or other work so that one setup can be used several times. Batching the work of the bottleneck is appropriate if some setup time is required at the bottleneck, because that setup time is nonproductive. Using the same setup several times in a row by batching the work minimizes the nonproductive portion of the day and maximizes production.

An inviting target for improvement at the bottleneck is to reduce setup time by bringing in new technology or perhaps by reorganizing the work. Reducing bottleneck setup time is good on its own because it reduces nonproductive time at the bottleneck.

Batching increases variability in the overall service performance time. Patients at the head of a batch are processed in less overall time than patients at the end of a batch; smaller batches are thus an indicator of improvements in overall system time.

Batching anywhere upstream or downstream is suspect. Because excess capacity exists everywhere other than at the bottleneck, reducing non-bottleneck setup time is not an obvious goal. As batching increases overall service time variability, it is probably a negative, except when it occurs at the bottleneck.

Bunching

Bunching is the unintentional grouping of patients or other work. Bunching is usually caused by others. Bunching is a surge of service demand or a surge of workflow into an activity. Dealing with that surge in demand requires resources.

Orthodontists serving the teenage market for braces face the fact that their demand will surge after school hours, and they figure that into their organization resource planning. British emergency departments can figure on a bunch of bleeding fans after major soccer matches.

Within the healthcare organization, bunching is an artifact of local optimization. For example, if the surgery department keeps all patients until the end of the shift and then sends them all to the postoperative patient care unit in a bunch, that may (or may not) be optimum for the surgery department, but it certainly presents the postoperative patient care unit with a surge of patients to handle. This may be the optimum policy for the organization, but it is suspect.

The pharmacy may deliver all medicine orders to a patient care unit in bunches, one or two times per shift, to reduce the cost of messengers and carts. This may be the right policy because it allows the patient care unit manager to focus on medicine at those few times per shift, and it probably does not change the overall medicine inventory level very much for the organization. The same is true for ordinary supply deliveries.

Bunching tends to increase the variability of overall service time and is therefore generally suspect. Bunching tends to require surge capacity and is suspect for that reason as well.

Hanging

Hanging, or hanging up, is waiting while some parallel process is completed. This may be as simple a matter as waiting for the delivery of routine supplies or waiting for an essential person required for the next task. Planning workflow in systems where hanging up is possible is tricky and usually requires planning in a wait time, which of course reduces capacity if the hanging up affects workflow through the bottleneck.

TIME-VALUE CHARTS

Consider the case of the patient who comes to a health service center for a diagnostic X-ray and advice from her doctor. Let us look at the timeline to see where value is being added and where no value is being added.

In exhibit 7.1, time proceeds to the right, and adding value causes the chart to grow upward. At the first step, the patient registers and presents personal information, which is a necessary part of the service and so adds value. Following that step is a wait, during which no value is added. The X-ray is then taken, which adds value. Then another wait occurs, which adds no value. The X-ray is interpreted by the doctor or doctors, and this adds value. A wait follows, which adds no value. A consultation is made with the patient, which adds value. Then another wait occurs, which adds no value. The bill is prepared, and this adds value. The patient then leaves, thereby completing the exercise.

Exhibit 7.1: Time-Value Chart for X-Ray Visit

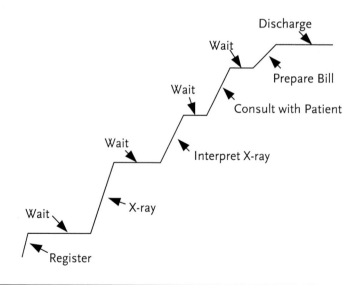

Note that the meaning of *value* here indicates an activity's value to the organization. The patient might be tempted to think that preparing the bill is not adding value (to her side of things), but of course it is from the organization's point of view. Note further that the value is being added by a variety of factors, including the patient, the admitting clerk, the X-ray technician, the medical doctors, the invoicing clerk, and perhaps others.

The vertical rise associated with each value-adding step is loosely proportional to the incremental value, but no particular precision is required. This is a sketch, not an accounting statement. The time lapses, on the other hand, should be tracked with some care because it is time that draws our attention here. The utility of a time-value chart is that the chart makes obvious where there are time lapses that do not add value. Getting rid of some of the gaps speeds up the overall service while not detracting at all from the value added.

A time-value chart is simple, yet it portrays much about the workings of the system. Why is each particular wait there? Why does each wait last as long as it does? What would be the benefit, if any, of reducing the wait? What is the cost to the organization of that wait? What is the cost to the patient, in lost time, for that wait?

The rules that govern workflow are necessarily management rules. Furthermore, they must be set at a senior management level to preclude one department from solving its problems by moving them to the next department. The senior management can issue rational workflow rules only if senior management understands where the bottleneck is, why it is there, and what the incentives are to keep the bottleneck flowing. Then, the senior management can develop and issue rules that govern flow through the bottleneck and through the upstream and downstream departments.

Senior management will also gain a basis for evaluating capital requests for the expansion of various departments. Will that capital expansion expand the bottleneck? If not, why is it being considered? Perhaps certain departments should be contracted to free up resources to expand the bottleneck.

BATCH OF ONE

From the point of view of the patient, the right batch size is one: the individual patient. In the patient's perfect scenario, there would be no waiting in queue at the MRI machine, no waiting for pending administrative actions, and no bunching up with other patients to suit the convenience of one service or another. This scenario would automatically be the case if batch-of-one were also the lowest-cost way of doing things for the healthcare organization. It is not yet so, but the trend is in that direction.

As more and more healthcare functions are computerized, mechanized, and even robotized, the incentive to batch patients goes down because, as the setup cost goes to zero, the most productive batch size goes to one.

In non-bottleneck departments, the batch size is arbitrary because plenty of slack is inherent by definition. In these departments, much could be done today to move in the direction of batch-of-one patient management.

At the bottleneck, where setup time needs to be spread across a batch of patients because setup time is a dead loss to the whole organization, capital investments to reduce setup time provide a twofold benefit. First, the productive capacity of the whole organization goes up. Second, the optimum batch size goes toward one, which pleases patients.

BOTTLENECK TRAFFIC CAPACITY ANALYSIS

Capacity analysis, the trade-off between capital investment and various measures of service level, has been modeled successfully using only very simple inputs for about a hundred years. The hero in this development was Anger Erlang, who was employed by the Copenhagen telephone company in the early part of the twentieth century. The question before him was how to establish capacity requirements for telephone lines while attaining some level of customer satisfaction.

It is remarkable that no breakthrough in the hundred years since then has displaced the Erlang statistical models, which are still used today to size telephone call centers as well as telephone lines and switches. Any finite capacity system doing discrete work can be analyzed with Erlang's statistical models.

This general field of study is called traffic engineering because the point of it all is to understand, manage, and design the system to serve the traffic. Erlang derived his models of telephone call traffic based on only these points: that calls are independent of each other, that the duration of any call may be longer or shorter but with some mean value, that a call not served immediately (blocked) may be dropped or kept in queue, and that only a small fraction of the total population will seek service in any time period.

From his theory, Erlang wrote statistical formulae for various matters, taking into account the factors that are of interest in capacity planning:

- The number of service units, such as MRI units or beds, providing the physical capacity
- The average service time measured in minutes, hours, or days
- The average count of new arrivals each minute, hour, or day

From these, two more items of interest are calculated:

- The traffic level, which is the product of average arrival count multiplied by the average service time
- The slack in the system, which is the fraction of capacity that is not used on average, over the time period of interest

There has to be some slack in the system if arrivals fluctuate at all. And there has to be some slack in the system over a longer period or else arrivals will simply stack up.

Erlang considered and developed statistical models for two situations: (1) Any arrival not served immediately goes away, and (2) arrivals not served immediately stay in a holding queue. Both are relevant to just about any service business.

Consider a nursing home that accepts patients discharged from a local hospital, and consider that there are several comparable nursing homes that compete for those patients. If the nursing home is full, then the next "arrival" is blocked and will go to another nursing home. No queue. How much slack should that nursing home plan for? Slack doesn't generate revenue, but on the other hand if there are rarely any beds available, the hospital will not bother to call. Perhaps the nursing home should plan to have one bed free 90 percent of the time. Erlang's no-queue analysis can inform nursing home management on how many extra physical beds, which is to say how much slack, would be required.

Exhibit 7.2 is an example; assume a fixed capacity of 30 beds and an average stay of seven days:

Exhibit 7.2: Likelihood of a Free Bed

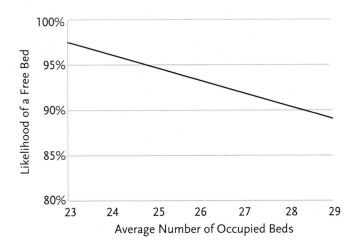

As the graph shows, to have a 90 percent likelihood of a free bed, the average occupancy has to be held at 28 patients. In other words, two beds have to be empty, on average, to be 90 percent confident of having at least one bed free.

Now consider an MRI center, and assume that there is no competing MRI center across the street so that patients will likely wait in queue rather than go elsewhere. It's good to have a few patients waiting in queue because that keeps the MRI machine humming. On the other hand, if lots of patients wait a long time in queue, word will get around and future patients will go elsewhere. What is a reasonable average wait time? What is the wait time that should not be exceeded for 90 percent of patients?

The management policy for the MRI center will probably dwell on the number of patients to book during the busy time of the day. How much busy-hour slack should be provided? No slack? Negative slack, thereby forcing patients into the queue? Ten percent slack? Lots of slack? Probably not lots of slack, unless a no-waiting price-adder can be realized. What would that price-adder have to be to make this a good policy? All of these policies can be analyzed with Erlang's statistical models. So can mixed traffic of scheduled patients and walk-in patients.

Erlang distributions can be expressed as combinations of Poisson distributions, which is handy because all spreadsheets provide Poisson functions (see appendix B). Cases later in the book provide hands-on opportunities to analyze the use of queuing and no-queuing in the nursing home and MRI center examples.

INTERRUPTIONS

Some interruptions are like a bolt from the blue, completely outside the range of experience.

Some interruptions are unlikely, but they are of such significance that hospitals go through drills to walk everyone through what can be expected in that unlikely occurrence. Perhaps a major flood or a tornado. Perhaps a mass-casualty event.

Most interruptions, though, are foreseeable, insofar as similar interruptions occurred in previous days or weeks. There is likely to be a notion or estimate or measure of how likely it is that the next interruption will be in the next hour or the next ten minutes.

Foreseeable Interruptions

Suppose experience shows that interruptions occur about once an hour. Counting from now, when will the next interruption occur? That question cannot be answered, but related questions can:

- How likely is it that there will be no interruptions in the next 5 minutes? Ninety percent.
- How likely is it that there will be no interruptions in the next 10 minutes? Eighty-five percent.
- How likely is it that there will be no interruptions in the next 20 minutes? Seventy-two percent.
- How likely is it that there will be no interruptions in the next 30 minutes? Sixty-one percent.
- How likely is it that there will be no interruptions in the next 40 minutes? Fifty-one percent.

If an essential task at hand takes 40 minutes to complete, it's even money that an interruption will occur before the essential task is completed.

To get down to a 15 percent likelihood of interruption, the essential task has to be reorganized so that the essential part is only, say, ten minutes long.

What to do? There are a few things to keep in mind:

- A completed task cannot be interrupted.
- An unstarted task cannot be interrupted.
- Time always counts from *now*.

So, study that 40-minute essential task to see what can be moved upstream or downstream and to see where hold points can be inserted to break the 40 minutes into, say, four 10-minute blocks separated by hold points.

Hold Points

Hold points are stable configurations—configurations such that the patient is not put in harm's way if an interruption occurs while holding, and from which work can be restarted in an orderly way.

Hold points can be used to verify that the prior task was successful, that any cleanup is complete, and that all documentation is up-to-date. Hold points should be used to preview the next task, to verify that all supplies are in hand, and to run through the checklist. If more than one person is involved, mutual review of who will be doing what is always in order, even if the same team does the same task fifty times a day. That's what pilots do. If the patient is conscious or the family is present, explaining what comes next is a good idea.

Foreseeable Branch Points

Dr. Atul Gawande (2004) has said that when sponges and tools get left behind by surgeons, it's almost always the case that the surgeon had begun expecting A but then discovered B. Call that a branch point, a particular sort of interruption in the flow of things. The possibility of B, or at least the likelihood of B, should be considered when the surgery is planned so that an orderly transition from A to B will transpire. This applies to all matters, not just surgery.

Roll Forward, Roll Back

If an interruption occurs during a critical period, the question is whether to continue the task as far as the next hold point (roll forward), or to stop the task and return to the prior hold point (roll back) if that is a meaningful choice. This needs to be thought through ahead of time.

Interruption at a Hold Point

Interruptions at hold points can be serviced, because that's the way the hold point is designed. Practice drills are helpful.

Reducing Interruptions

While there are plenty of interruptions that arise outside anyone's control, there are others that can be reduced or eliminated. For instance, an IV pump with two fluid pouches and the ability to switch from one to the other requires the same number of replenishments per shift, but the timing is less critical.

Professor Tucker has reported extensively on a case where a nurse, coming to bedside, discovered that the room's hand sanitizer dispenser was empty (Tucker and Spear 2006). That introduced a delay, and then something else happened and then something else, and then. . . . The result was that the nurse never did get that patient-care task done. Well, hanging two hand-sanitizer dispensers in each room might not break the bank. Ditto paper towels, disposable gloves, and so on. That is to say, policy might well indicate that supplies should be provisioned so that time-critical events never arise. Running out of such supplies should be a never event. Getting to "never" in this case means that the housekeeping department needs to embrace room-provisioning as essential to patient safety, something more than just one more thing to get done along with mopping the floors.

DISTRACTIONS

Noise, lights, public address announcements, and computer beeps and messages are distractions that contribute to stress and sensory overload. Computer matters are dealt with in chapter 8. The others, which can perhaps be called work-environment distractions, need to be dealt with by a redesign of the workplace.

If staff tune the distractions out, there is a high risk that an important message will get lost in the clutter, the message getting tuned out along with the noise. Such distractions wear on patients and family, too, and perhaps more so, because patients and family will have no basis for sorting out important messages from the clutter.

Computerization of Healthcare

Computerization is coming on fast, moving from data-logging to autonomous patients and autonomous machines. While some old problems have gone away, some brand new ones have sprung up, such as data overload. There are lessons to be learned from other industries.

PRIMARY LESSONS

Industry—in particular High-Reliability Organizations—have learned the following lessons through mistakes and misfortunes. Sooner or later, healthcare will learn these lessons, too. Might as well learn them now, for free.

1. *Control data entry.* The old saying "garbage in, garbage out" has been replaced with a new formulation: Take the time and effort to make sure only valid data get into the records, because the cost of catching up with and fixing errors grows exponentially thereafter.
2. *Clean up the system,* then *computerize.* A system that has flaws will have the same flaws when computerized, only the flaws will occur much faster. It is not unusual to set out to clean up a system so that computers can be introduced, only to find that the cleaned-up system doesn't need computers at all.
3. *Any computer will fail at the awkward moment.* Often, this failure will take a process in an unsafe direction. We must protect the patient from the computer.

4. *Know the state of the system.* When something dreadful happens, look for the computer-system operator who does not know the state of the system and does not know what the computer is doing (Reason 1990). The remedy for this is better human factors engineering. This is a very difficult problem, probably the most difficult problem in any computerized industry and particularly in healthcare right now.

This book considers each of these topics from the Six Sigma perspective, which calls for proper task design, proper communications, and proper assignment of responsibility.

Computerization is a boon to High-Reliability Organizations and will be a boon to healthcare. Computerization is not trivial and takes quite a lot of adjustment in traditional thinking and processes. Healthcare is only at the beginning of the computerization phase, two or three generations behind High-Reliability Organizations. Lessons are available for the learning.

ELECTRONIC PATIENT RECORDS AND DATA ENTRY

Nearly all hospitals have electronic patient records now, and a fraction of independent physicians' offices do. Over the next few years, it seems likely that nearly all doctors will be added to the electronic patient records, and then others will join, eventually bringing in everyone who is, say, licensed to write a prescription, such as dentists.

The quality of the information in the electronic patient records (Nerny 2015) is open to question. Given American experience with other large databases—the Social Security Administration, for example, identifies 6.5 million citizens as being 112 years old (Associated Press 2015)—the fraction of electronic patient records with serious errors is probably around 20 percent. No large study of this matter in patient records has been reported.

In any database, it is very difficult to keep up with and correct errors after the data are entered. The best practice is to focus on keeping inadvertent error from putting bum data in.

To address inadvertent error in the data-entry task, follow the three Six Sigma rules: design the task to make the task more likely to succeed than to fail, make any error obvious to the data-entry person, and make it easy to correct errors on the spot, before bum data get into the database.

There are good examples of low-error data entry. Consider online shopping. The shopper selects some items and clicks a button. A page opens up showing a summary of the order for the shopper to review and to correct quantities, delete unwanted items, back up, cancel the whole thing, or finish the purchase. In computer jargon, this is a two-phase commit. The first phase gathers the data but keeps the data well away from the database; the second phase changes the database by making the new entries.

Better shopping sites hold the order for a period so that the shopper can consider the matter further, intercept, and reverse the order even after the "buy" button has been clicked. If the order is intercepted, then the database is rolled back to its prior state. After that grace period, if there is no interception, the database is rolled forward to recognize the order, and the fulfillment and billing wheels begin to turn.

To apply this to patient records, consider the nurse at the bedside who scans the patient's ID badge and the nurse's own ID badge, takes vital signs, performs other actions, and makes entries into a computer. Before the nurse leaves the bedside, the computer should open a page with a summary of the nurse's entries and present buttons to confirm or correct entries. Perhaps the page should highlight unusual entries such as a new drug for this patient, an override of a barcode scan, or other departures from normal.

Pamela Peele, analytics chief for the insurance division of UPMC in Pittsburgh, is quoted as saying, "You're not going to get stand-up analytics if you don't have data fit for consumption. Groom it up and you immediately get cost savings" (Morse 2016).

Data can be wrong in a patient record for reasons other than data-entry errors, as discussed in the "Intrinsic Variability" section later in this chapter.

OTHER USES OF ELECTRONIC PATIENT RECORDS, OTHER DATABASES

Mass studies of electronic patient records, which would simply have been impossible to do with paper records, show patient-flow and patient-care patterns such as excess returns to the operating room, changes in medication, early return to the hospital after discharge, and the like (Lieber 2015). Unexpected patterns may draw attention to matters that can be improved. These studies are an unanticipated benefit of electronic patient records.

There is another database that provides information on a particular set of patients: those involved in litigation. PIAA's (2016) Data Sharing Project, available at www.piaa.us, is a medical malpractice database that is available to the public for study and helps find markers that might have made a difference in these troubling cases.

BIG DATA

Consider the universe of Internet queries. Microsoft has studied the queries entered into the Microsoft Bing search engine by people who later exhibited pancreatic cancer (Paparrizos, White, and Horvitz 2016). The queries show a pattern, as these people started wondering and querying about symptoms they discovered in themselves. Given that this particular cancer has a high mortality rate, perhaps it is worth asking if these self-revealing queries constitute a marker that should trigger early intervention.

In this case, it is the Bing query engine itself that "knows" who is performing the queries. What should Bing do? Send a note to that person? Send the person's name to a drug manufacturer? Or to the person's primary care physician, if that could be determined? Perhaps enter the information into the electronic patient record, if possible?

Google (2016) developed a flu-tracking system that shows flu outbreaks on a map. This is not specific to a person but rather is epidemiological, based on query patterns. The Google report was shown to be about the same as the government's CDC report, but *two weeks earlier*, a phenomenon that has come to be called *now-casting*. The Google report generated a great deal of controversy because Google uses search patterns only, with no underlying medical or epidemiological mechanism. Google has suspended publication of the flu tracker presently, and access is restricted to academic researchers. Now-casting, though, is certainly here to stay. Consider the public health value of now-casts, which can guide timely vaccine shipments, as opposed to historical patterns, which cannot.

INTRINSIC VARIABILITY

Six Sigma emphasizes getting rid of controllable variability, such as data-entry errors, so that intrinsic variability can be observed and perhaps reduced by system redesign.

One point of intrinsic variability in electronic patient records is final diagnosis. Autopsy studies show that pre-death diagnoses are wrong 8 percent of the time when the final diagnosis is made in a hospital with labs and machines all around, and 40 percent of the time when the final diagnosis is made in a doctor's office (Lieber 2015). Note that there is no assertion that the diagnoses were made in error; rather, this is the best result that current diagnostic methods can achieve. This variability is intrinsic presently. In the future, studies may reveal markers that would allow better diagnoses, and the studies can proceed with greater confidence if the controllable variability, such as data-entry error, is greatly reduced.

The parallels between autopsy/diagnoses studies and the Microsoft study cited earlier are informative.

MESSAGE OVERLOAD AND THE TIME BASIS FOR COMPUTER-TO-PERSON COMMUNICATIONS

Doctors can and often now do enter orders on smartphones using specialized apps and secure connections. The computer on the receiving end sends the order forward for action, makes an entry in the patient's record, and sends back an acknowledgment to the doctor. In addition, entries made by other parties are reported back to the doctor's phone.

Concerns arise now that messages flowing back to the doctor's smartphone have become overwhelming in number and frequency, to the extent that serious messages are lost in a blizzard (Luthra 2016). The app vendors are being told to develop filters to reduce the quantity of messages by suppressing the "less important" ones (Luthra 2016). That might work, but it will always be open to challenge because the software, rather than the doctor, would be in control.

Here's another approach: Rather than letting each event trigger a message, consider time-base messaging.

The idea is that, while computers can generate a million messages per second, a more workable way is to consider time from the patient's point of view. What is a reasonable frequency, from the patient's point of view, for the doctor to receive a message, consider what to do, and issue a new order if a new order is deemed necessary? Once an hour? Twice an hour? Twenty times an hour?

Suppose that, for a particular patient, twice an hour is judged by the doctor to be a prudent response time. In that case, messages to the doctor for this patient can be collected over 30 minutes, summarized, and sent as one message.

For another patient, ten-minute updates might be in order. For another, once a day.

The upshot is that the doctor is being informed in a timely manner for each patient, more frequently for selected patients and less frequently for others, without a blizzard of messages.

Urgent events can still trigger an immediate message with an appropriate urgent-sounding ringtone.

Time-base messaging derives from the thinking of Carnegie Mellon University (CMU)'s Allen Newell, one of the founders of modern computer science. Newell asked himself if a computer should respond as quickly as possible to an event, and he decided against this because to do so would keep the computer busy to

Allen Newell

Newell (1927–1992) was
a researcher in computer
science and cognitive
psychology at RAND
Corporation and CMU. In
1975, Newell was a joint
winner of the Turing Award
with Nobel laureate Herbert
A. Simon, and in 1989 he was
named a William James Fellow
by the American Psychological
Society (now called the
Association for Psychological
Science).

no benefit to the outside world. Rather, a reasonable response time would suffice while reducing the burden on the computer. In the application we just discussed, Newell's thinking is reversed to reduce the burden on the human.

Alarm overload and alarm fatigue arise in the operating room and elsewhere in healthcare (Solet and Barach 2012). Time-base messaging can help there, too.

AUTONOMY AND PATIENT SAFETY

Computerization in healthcare started with bookkeeping, important but a long way from the patient.

Computerized patient records came later and, if in error, can misinform a caregiver who might take an action that puts the patient in harm's way. However, the caregiver stands between the patient record and the patient, and the caregiver is trained to be prudent. The caregiver does not give over control to the electronic record.

Computerized order entry can put the patient in harm's way by accepting a drug order that is too high by a factor of ten, say. In this case, the action is in plain view of the doctor who will catch errors and correct them on the spot. The doctor does not give over control to the order-entry computer.

Presently, computers keep records and execute orders in plain view, no transfer of control. But soon, computers will have substantial autonomy to take action.

Consider HIFU (Kennard 2016), which stands for high-intensity, focused ultrasound, a computerized treatment for certain cancers of the prostate. This is an important development, providing noninvasive treatment for, potentially, a very large population of aging men. HIFU starts with computer analysis of magnetic resonance imaging (MRI) data and proceeds to computer-controlled obliteration of tiny clusters of cancer cells by focusing several high-intensity ultrasound sources so that the beams cross at the right point in the patient's prostate. After the treatment, the patient wakes up, gets dressed, and walks out the door. No diapers, no side effects. Amazing.

The HIFU treatment can only be done by computer because the multiple, precise actions are beyond what a human can do. The urologist can watch with keen interest, but that's about all. There's a STOP button, but otherwise the computer is autonomous.

Now suppose the HIFU computer makes a mistake. Wrong focus target? Some healthy tissue is lost but the patient's safety is not compromised.

Computers are fallible. Prudent design, as practiced by High-Reliability Organizations, postulates that the computer will fail at the awkward moment, that the computer will fail in the worst possible way, *and* that the computer cannot correct itself or take safety-first actions on its own.

For autonomous computers, something outside the computer must ensure patient safety. Usually that means a separate, freestanding computer that takes the necessary actions to override the autonomous computer to protect the patient's safety. This is called "separation of control and protection" in other industries. Perhaps "separation of autonomy from patient safety" might be a better name for this rule when it is applied in healthcare.

This is only a concern for those cases where control of what's going on passes from the human to the computer. So long as the human is in control, the human should be able to keep matters in hand and keep the patient out of harm's way.

HIFU technology has now been approved by the US Food and Drug Administration to treat a certain tremor by ablating brain cells under MRI and computer control (FDA 2016). Other applications will surely follow. The same concerns of control and protection arise.

Not all medical robots are involved in patient care directly. Consider the very useful Xenex robot that operates autonomously to sanitize a patient's room after discharge. This is very important for patient safety. Nosocomial infections are a leading mechanism for patient harm (Xenex 2016).

THE EVOLVED IV POLE

Consider the IV pole. In primal form, the IV pole is a pole that dispenses fluid from a pouch, which is hung from a hook high enough up that the fluid flows downhill to the patient.

Now, advance its technology:

◆ Add a pump so that the fluid flows at a precise rate.
◆ Add a second hook and pouch, and tell the pump to switch to the second pouch when the first one is exhausted.
◆ Add a barcode scanner so that the pump will "know" what fluid is in each pouch.
◆ Add a network interface so that the pump can report to the patient's record, to the pharmacy, and to the nurse's station for each event and can trigger alarms if both pouches run dry.

That's the state of the art at this writing. The IV pump is running by itself but is not autonomous.

Now, consider the *near* future:

- Add software so that the pump orders new pouches from the pharmacy itself in a timely manner, providing the room and bed number.
- Add software to make the replenishment order by medication, perhaps sending the barcode of the current pouches.
- Add software to order replenishment by "reading" the patient's record and standing orders.
- Add software and a bit of hardware so that the pump dismounts old pouches and mounts new ones after checking barcodes.

Now consider the errors the pump might make in each of these autonomous actions. Wrong bed number? What happens? Wrong barcode? What happens? Wrong reading of the patient's record? What happens?

While the first impulse is to build checks into the software, the Six Sigma design rule stipulates that the protective action must be separate from the autonomous computer controlling the process.

So long as a human is mounting the pouches, the human can be instructed to verify barcodes, validate against standing orders, and so on. The human protects the patient.

But if the computer is mounting the pouches with no human in sight, what needs to be added, separate from the autonomous computer? Perhaps a separate device with a barcode reader and sufficient, separately entered information to approve or thwart the mounting action, with some alarms.

While the self-pouch-mounting IV pump exists a bit in the future, there are plenty of computerized medical devices that are close to the line. Ventilators, to take one simple example, can cause patient death if even a single knob is set wrong. Where is the separate protection there?

WEARABLES

The term wearables covers smartphones, smart wrist straps, smart wristwatches, and now "smart Band-Aids" (Rhythm Diagnostic Systems 2016), all of which have built-in sensors that communicate wirelessly with computers. Wearables are evolving rapidly and are already changing the way people manage their healthcare.

As costs continue to fall, the devices will become ubiquitous, and the traditional model of healthcare management will shift in ways not yet known.

There is an official name for wearables: *medical body area networks*, or MBANs. Maybe that term will catch on. The Federal Communications Commission (FCC) has allocated separate spectrum for MBANs in addition to spectrum already designated for communications having a medical/industrial/scientific use and a collection of specific medical-related applications. The FCC is stingy with spectrum, so this is an important addition (Slabodkin 2016).

Today, smartphones can perform eye-chart tests and hearing acuity tests, take the pulse rate, and read out the blood-oxygen saturation level, all while keeping track of location and movement. Smart wrist straps and smart wristwatches do the same. They all accumulate data and generate reports, telling the wearer how many steps were taken today, how much time was spent recumbent, and so on. Some devices perform sleep analysis. All use Bluetooth or equivalent wireless technology to pair with a cell phone and communicate with the whole world via the Internet.

The immediate next wave in MBANs is the smart Band-Aid. Consider a paste-on strip equipped with tiny sensors, a tiny computer, and a tiny Bluetooth radio. The sensors detect movement and measure temperature on the skin surface. Affix more smart Band-Aids on different spots on the body, get more data. The smart Band-Aid can already measure at least the following:

- Pulse, pulse wave, and changes thereof
- Respiration rate and changes thereof
- Chest sounds, knee sounds, and the like
- Fetal heart rate
- Temperature hot spots and cold spots, which are important for the feet of diabetic patients
- Sleep cycles
- Footsteps and irregularity in gait
- Combinations of these, such as a change in respiration rate after climbing stairs
- Falls and missteps
- Location and departure from a prescribed area

A very large number of people—perhaps millions—know how to program applications, or apps, for smartphones. The emergence of smart Band-Aids will trigger a whole new wave of apps, such as eye-movement tests that determine whether a dizzy person has had a stroke. Figure, too, that these apps will feed wearable data to medical diagnostics websites, particularly if the person's medical history is in hand.

Who will be in control of and have access to the wearable data? The person in question, surely. Family members? The family doctor? How the data generated by wearables will fit into the overall scheme of things is yet to be known. Will data be fed to existing patient electronic records or to third-party data vaults? Who owns the wearable data? How will wearable data be validated and verified before they get into records? How will bad data be purged?

An enhanced version of the smart Band-Aid can now perform an EKG. Even smart sutures are not far off (Kulbatski 2016). These futuristic threads do all the temperature- and displacement-sensing and reporting the smart Band-Aids do, and more. Smart sutures perform biological analysis, including measuring pH and glucose levels, and report their results wirelessly. The first practical applications are likely to monitor wound healing and the integration of surgically implanted orthopedics and organs—and who knows what else?

There are also a great many medical gadgets (Bennett 2012) that plug into iPhones and other types of smartphones: Otoscope. EKG. Microscope. Glucometer. Dermatoscope. Forehead thermometer. Ultrasound. Petri dish. Slit lamp. Blood pressure cuff. Spirometer. Breathalyzer. That's today. More are coming. These devices aren't quite wearables—yet. They are, however, intended for at-home use by the general public, either on their own or in partnership with a doctor, who is automatically sent the data generated by the device.

One of the hopes is that wearables will bring a new interest in self-directed medical care. Some limited studies show that persons who are involved with monitoring themselves are more apt to adhere to instructions. Perhaps wearables will increase a patient's adherence to a doctor's orders for medication use, exercise, and diet.

THE PATIENT'S ADVOCATE

The literature advises taking somebody with you when you go to the hospital, somebody who will know what's going on, ask questions, check badges, challenge medications, keep you from falling out of bed, and keep visitors from sitting on the bed. That's great, if such a person exists (PAO 2016).

The Patient's Advocate movement is the human analog to protecting the patient from the computer. The Patient's Advocate movement assumes that the whole healthcare system, however well meaning, will fail at the awkward moment.

Consider a patient in a hospital bed, with people coming and going throughout the day and night. What would the ideal Patient's Advocate do? When the room door opens and somebody comes in, the Advocate speaks up:

"Hello," the Advocate says. "Are you here for Mrs. Elizabeth Jones of Baskerville?

"State your name and show me your badge, please.

"Tell me why you are here, please.

"You are a visitor? Please smile for the camera and state your name. You'll find a hand-sanitizer dispenser next to the door. Please don't sit on the bed.

"Show me the label and barcode on that medicine, please. I think that is a new medication. Can you please show me the doctor's order?

"Show me the dietary order for that food tray, please.

"Please show me the order to take Mrs. Jones to X-ray.

"I'm sorry to mention this, Doctor, but I am required to remind you to wash your hands and your stethoscope.

"Do you have any new instructions for Mrs. Jones?

"Thank you."

A modern smartphone can do all those things: Detect motion when the door opens and when people move about. Read barcodes. Recognize voices. Understand basic speech in any language. Match face images. Record events, timeline, audio, video. Be alert at all hours. Call for help.

It's time for the Patient's Advocate app.

If the smartphone has access to patient information, preferably information independent of the hospital's records, then the smartphone app can cross-check medications against allergies, and so on, doing a bit more to protect the patient.

Can a smartphone keep a patient from falling when getting out of bed? A smartphone plus one or two smart Band-Aids can know immediately when the patient starts to sit up or move legs in a way that reveals an intention to get out of bed. The smartphone can then say, "Mrs. Jones, please stay in bed. The nurses' station has been notified that you need help, and someone is coming. Can you wait just a few minutes, please? Can you tell me what you want to do? Maybe I can help you."

Change Management

Improving the system will require changes to be made. However, the changes should first be tried out on some small scale so that lessons can be learned without risking the whole of the organization.

SELECTING CHANGES

The first thing to be decided when making changes is whether you want to make many small ones or a few big ones. The following pages will address some of the positive and negative aspects of both routes.

MANY SMALL CHANGES

C. Edwards Deming, when advising companies in post–World War II Japan, recommended that everyone participate in making changes, on the basis that the worker is the important element and that letting the worker improve processes is key. This is the "hurdle" notion: Workers would be more successful if hurdles were removed, and who knows better what the hurdles are than the actual worker? A small group of workers or the small team of workers from various departments will know and identify the hurdles.

Quality Circles

In the 1980s, many American firms experimented with *quality circles*, an idea imported from Japan. A quality circle is a group of employees—not managers—drawn from adjacent departments who select a small improvement to be made. They make this improvement by drawing small amounts of money from the organization as might be needed to carry the work out. These quality circles seemed to do some good and very little harm, and they were an interesting experiment in industrial group dynamics. However, American interest in them seems to have waned in recent years. The improvements were almost guaranteed to work because those involved in making them work were the very same people who sponsored the improvement.

Quality circles were generally operated on lunch breaks and were "unmanaged," so the cost to the organization was small. In Japan, quality circles commonly meet in the evening, on noncompany time. Quality circles are one way of getting to Deming's ideal, but other ways also are available.

Campaigns

A campaign is another way of getting lots of smaller things done. In a campaign, one particular goal is set, and everybody is encouraged to meet it by the end of the month or day. Crosby favors "zero defect day" campaigns. Walmart features pep rallies for its associates who work on the store floor. These are one-day-at-a-time campaigns. Although many people find such campaigns annoying, distracting, unprofessional, and not at all motivating, the fact is that some people respond to campaigns very positively. Varsity athletes are given pep talks and immediate goals to reach (win the game, score the goal, hit the ball). Because these athletes have been hearing the same pep talks since they were eight years old, they are conditioned to respond with increased concentration and effort. Sales departments run on campaigns, with those who meet the special monthly sales goal winning a steak dinner or a trip to Hawaii. All sales departments run campaigns, and all salespeople are motivated to concentrate all the harder to meet their goals; it is therefore not surprising to find that many companies go out of their way to hire varsity athletes to work in their sales departments.

Suggestion Boxes

Mandatory suggestion boxes are a different sort of campaign, with the same campaign being repeated again and again. Employees are exhorted to turn in suggestions for improvement of the workplace or the products. Because they are exhorted, they feel some pressure to think up something to suggest; this gets the employees' heads involved in the game at least for a long enough time to think of some new idea. Some Japanese companies, with very gentle exhortation, get hundreds of suggestions per month *per employee*. The likelihood that any of these will be red-hot suggestions is small, but if the purpose is to keep the employee thinking about the job, mandatory suggestion plans will likely meet that goal. On the other hand, a passive suggestion box, lacking the exhortation, is likely to occupy the mind of few employees.

Whether active or passive, suggestion boxes take up some management time and therefore have a cost because somebody has to read the suggestions and potentially prepare a response to the originator. Japanese companies seem to like their mandatory suggestion box system. American and European firms that are pleased with their passive suggestion boxes seem to be few in number.

FEWER, LARGER CHANGES

Juran (1995) favors undertaking fewer, larger changes. In fact, Juran goes so far as to say that only those changes that pose a breakthrough potential—something of great commercial value—should be undertaken at all. This is an extreme position, but extreme positions can help clarify thinking.

The fact that management is already busy argues in favor of making few changes at a time. Any significant project will require management attention. Any project crossing organizational lines will take more management attention, and significant projects will likely cross organizational lines in a healthcare organization because of the way the work flows through the organization. Nontrivial projects require funding for capital equipment and expenses, even at the trial stage. This necessarily involves management.

Changes almost always have unforeseen ripple effects. These ripple effects may be positive or negative; one hopes for the positive. In either case, the ripples have to be looked after and understood. Gaining this understanding is not likely if several projects are causing ripples at the same time.

Other things are also going on in the organization that must be taken into consideration, such as equipment updates, facility renovations, managers' promotions, the additions of new treatments, new regulations being promulgated by various agencies, and new employees being hired to respond to turnover and growth. These all demand management attention as well as resources, and management can only do so much.

THE CHOICE OF MANY VERSUS FEW

The many-versus-few choice is up to the organization's senior management. We personally recommend fewer projects, because we find the Juran argument persuasive on balance and solicitous of the management burden.

If the choice is made to go with a few projects, how will you know which ones are most necessary? Experience shows that the senior management knows where the problems are because they hear about them all the time. The senior group may not know what the problem is exactly, and they are not at all likely to have useful quantitative information in hand. However, they do know where the problems are because everybody tells them. The senior management group could make a pretty good list of projects just by polling their own group. Indeed, Juran recommends exactly this. This process gets right to the point.

Management may choose to invite midlevel management to participate in project targeting or may invite a cross-section of management and professional staff. This decision is a question of local management style, and there is merit in maintaining consistency in this arena. High-Reliability Organizations favor all-levels participation and deference to experts.

THINKING THROUGH THE PROPOSAL

One of the formulations of Murphy's Law (Murphy 1949) is that nature sides with the hidden flaw. Thinking through any proposed trial change includes thinking about the things that can go wrong by drawing on experience, the knowledge of the staff and the institution, and their collective knowledge about the particular change. This is known as *potential problem analysis*.

The point of this type of analysis is to anticipate the ripple effects that the potential change being considered may cause and to determine if the change should be modified or extended in some way to head off the ripples. Consider exhibit 9.1, which examines the things that might go wrong with a mail cart that has a new wheel design. What potential problems come with a new wheel design? Some possibilities are that the new wheel design may not work or that the wheel might come off or break.

The chart helps focus attention on what problems might arise and helps decision makers think through any mitigating actions that ought to be incorporated or any modifications to the proposed change that should be made. The chart may bring out some particular matters that ought to be tested specifically during the trial period.

Exhibit 9.1: Example of a Potential Problem Analysis

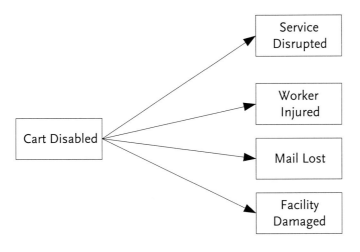

Potential problem analysis is simple enough in practice and is generally found to be worthwhile if kept to a suitable level of detail.

THE NATURE OF TRIALS

If management had had all the quantitative information in hand in an organized way with clear implications identified, it would have made the change a long time ago. Now, they likely begin with a general notion of what to do and where to do it but without a quantified basis for making the decision. Therefore, the way to proceed is to quantify the baseline, design a change, try it out in a small way, look hard at the outcome, quantify the results, and decide whether to extend the change to the whole organization. The trial may be localized to one group doing one activity, but it is more likely to be a trial along one workflow set of activities.

Gathering information to characterize the existing system is necessarily the first step so the results of the trial can be compared with something in a quantitative way. Once the existing system is suitably characterized, the trial can be designed with specific goals written down. The trial is then carried out, and both the data anticipated in the trial design and the unexpected data (ripples), which caused management, in its wisdom, to test the change in trial size in the first place, are gathered.

With the trial data in hand, a reasoned recommendation can be made to accept or reject the change. Except in trivial cases, some uncertainty will surround that recommendation. Analysis can quantify this, but it cannot eliminate it. The final decision to accept or reject the change rests with management.

The Participants Decide the Outcome

Most people are happy to participate in a trial. They figure it might be fun, and if it works they can brag about their participation later. If it fails, they will at least have stories to tell on bowling night. These folks can be counted on to give it a try, figure out little adjustments to make the change work better, and give straight feedback to the project leader.

However, those who are threatened by the trial are unlikely to be helpful in carrying it out, no matter how remote the threat. How threatened people feel has very little to do with what is said to them when the trial starts and much more to do with how the organization has behaved in comparable situations in the past. If the organization has a sorry track record in this regard, that is hard to overcome in one trial or even ten.

People can also be expected to be hostile toward the trial if it is perceived as an evaluation of *them* rather than of the work or workflow. To the extent that the trial shows that some people are making errors and the trial highlights those errors, it may well be concluded that the trial is a test of the workers themselves. What to do?

The answer is to make sure the trial is interpreted as a test of the *system* and not of the *people*. If a person is performing a task incorrectly, that is not a failing of the person, it is a failing of the system that did not teach that person how to complete the task.

However, how does the system treat people who are not correctly trained? Does the supervisor chastise the worker with a birch switch? Does the supervisor ask the worker if retraining is in order or if the task setup is wrong? Does the supervisor post control charts or their equivalent without names and let workers ask for retraining? Does retraining put the person's job at risk? Do workers even know if they are performing the task correctly? Does the system punish mistakes, thereby encouraging them to be hidden?

It is easy to say—and Deming says it—that the workers must believe the issue is always with the system, not with themselves. Furthermore, the workers must believe that management believes it. Deming goes further, saying that workers should never be given performance appraisals because these are given based on the notion that the person can do something to improve his or her own performance, which Deming believes goes against the "it is the system that is deficient" model.

Whether many organizations get to the Deming state is not known and seems unlikely. However, in the healthcare field, much of the service rests with professionals who are self-motivated in the first place and may come reasonably close to being Deming's model employees. These professionals set the tone for the whole organization. If the professionals are supportive of trials and of change, the organization has a reasonable shot at getting fair results from any trial.

Whether or not performance appraisals are used, management must review its evaluation process for *supervisors* to make sure nothing in the trial is antithetical to the interests of the supervisors of the work activity. If a supervisor is being evaluated and rewarded on the basis of moving patients through an activity as quickly as possible, and if the trial involves slowing patients down to prevent overloading the next location, something has to give. All such incentives and disincentives need to be considered in the design of any change to the system; potential problem analysis applies.

With that in mind, the trial is run in this obvious process:

1. Send out a draft to get comments beforehand.
2. Walk everybody through it.
3. Train anybody who needs training.
4. Track the data, share the data, post the data.
5. Watch for exceptions, hidden defects in the plan, and employee response. Walk around and listen to people.
6. Do not jump to premature conclusions. Get enough data and take enough time.
7. Be dispassionate.
8. Be ready to kill the trial if things do not work out.
9. Take notes. This education is expensive.

In-Trial Data Gathering

The trial will have specific objectives that can be quantified beforehand. Any one activity will have only two characteristic parameters: the average value and the standard deviation. The trial intends to move one of these, or perhaps both, but that is all it can hope to do.

Data gathering proceeds as follows:

1. The baseline control charts are in hand.
2. New control charts will be provided at the start of the trial showing where the data points are expected to fall.

3. Data are gathered and logged in the new control charts.
4. Exceptions, trends, and general behavior are examined throughout the trial.
5. Anecdotal information is logged as well; not everything can be reduced to numbers.
6. Decision points (off-ramps) are planned into the trial schedule. The trial leader reports to management at each of these times with a recommendation to proceed or to kill the trial.

The Bathtub Curve

The bathtub curve looks like a bathtub: high on one end, low in the middle, and high on the other end. The bathtub curve is a good representation of what very often happens in a trial, whether the trial involves machinery, people, or both.

In general, a machine's lifetime follows the bathtub curve. Some infant mortalities occur in the beginning, as computer equipment is particularly prone to infant mortality. This is followed by a long period during which everything works fine. Then, finally, failures happen again when the machines start wearing out.

Curiously, people show the same sort of curve. At the beginning, mistakes are made while people are getting the hang of the new procedure. Then a long period passes when the skills are being applied with little conscious effort, and then there is a period of increasing error, when bad habits creep in.

Because these are such common characteristics, any trial can be expected to reveal them. As the trial begins, productivity and service may be worse than before while people and equipment get adapted to the new scheme. Too-early evaluation of the trial may give a false-negative outcome. Evaluation during the period when work is going smoothly may give a false-positive outcome. Then in the final period, workers are getting a little sloppy, and evaluation at this period may give a false-negative outcome.

Numbers

Numbers are important, but they are not everything. Collecting anecdotes, feelings, and impressions is important, too.

When is it *safe* to evaluate the trial? It is never entirely safe, because there will always be some risk of reading the results incorrectly. On the basis of the numbers, however, this can be quantified into a level of confidence that the right interpretation is being made. On the basis of the management of people, some judgment is required.

To complete the bathtub analogy, the third phase, when errors are on the upswing, invites the replacement of worn hardware and the retraining of people (see exhibit 9.2). The most conservative trials run well into this third phase so that machine maintenance and retraining can be evaluated as part of the trial. However, this is too conservative for most organizations.

Exhibit 9.2: Example of a Bathtub Curve

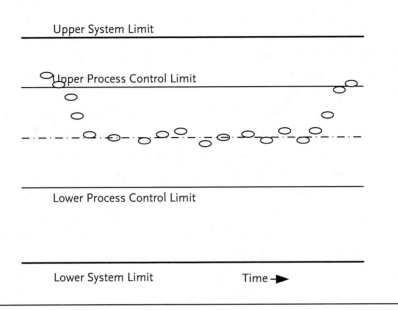

A mathematical distribution function actually exists that represents the bathtub curve; it is called the *Weibull function*, in honor of its inventor. Excel even incorporates it as a built-in function, WEIBULL.DIST(. . .).

The Null Hypothesis

Each trial will be designed to test whether a beneficial effect is gained. Because the old system had some variability and because the new system will have some variability, it is important that the trial be designed in such a way that the analyst can tell from the trial's data whether the effect is really there.

The designer of the trial poses a hypothesis. Suppose the analyst says, "The new average X-ray delivery time will be reduced by 20 minutes." This seems to be a sensible proposition, and gathering data about X-ray delivery times would likely provide a basis for evaluating the progress. There would be some variability, and that is to be expected.

To apply the tools of statistics to the evaluation of progress, it is necessary to cast the hypothesis in a form that statistics can address. This requires the application of a certain logic; this is done not because the logic is overwhelmingly attractive on its own merit but rather because it is the only logic that statisticians currently know how to analyze. Statistics is only about a hundred years old, making it one of the youngest branches of mathematics; compare that with the geometry books that still do things the way Euclid did. Perhaps, in the next hundred years, a more appealing approach to the analysis of hypotheses will arise.

To apply the tools of statistics, the starting point is the *null hypothesis*. The null hypothesis states that there is no change. In our X-ray delivery case, the null hypothesis posits that the average delivery time will be unchanged. The outcome of the trial will be one of two possibilities: the null hypothesis is supported or the null hypothesis is rejected.

However, allowance must be made for variability and uncertainty. Rather than a flat-out statement of support or rejection, the outcome will be stated with a certain degree of confidence, say 90 percent. The outcome will be stated, "With 90 percent confidence, the null hypothesis is supported (or rejected)."

Two special cases should be considered. Suppose the data support the conclusion that the null hypothesis is to be rejected when in fact the underlying truth is that it should be supported. This is called a *false-negative* outcome. The opposite can also happen, and this is called a *false-positive* outcome. Both are of concern in the design and evaluation of any trial. It is not correct to jump to the conclusion that if the null hypothesis is not supported, the hypothesis must be accepted. There is a gray area where the data can support neither a positive nor a negative conclusion.

At the data analysis level, all trials boil down to being either a null-hypothesis test of the average value of a distribution or a null-hypothesis test of the standard deviation of a distribution, or perhaps both at the same time. Statistical analysis can only deal with these limited, numeric concepts. If statistical analysis is to be applied, the analyst must cast the trial into these limited terms.

Trial Duration

If the trial is to determine the reliability of a laboratory instrument having a mean-time-to-failure of five years, the trial is going to take a very long time. If the trial has to do with a medical event that is shown in historical records to happen once every month or so, the trial is going to take a number of months; if it is carried out for a shorter time than that, nobody is going to believe the result.

How much data will be enough? If the data are easy to get and are generated in huge quantities every day, the question is not very important. More data always support a clearer conclusion, so get more data if they are free. Unhappily, free and easily obtainable data are rarely found in the real world. Getting data takes time and effort, so knowing how much data will be required is a necessary part of the trial design process. Because time goes by while the data are being collected, having an idea of how many data samples are required bears directly on how long the trial will take.

The answer to the question "How much data do we need?" depends on the confidence level required. If the confidence level is set at 75 percent, calculating a minimum data set size is possible. If the confidence level is set at 90 percent, more data will be needed, and if the confidence level is set at 95 percent, it will require more data still.

No absolute rule exists on what confidence level to set, but here are some general guidelines:

♦ Pick 75 percent if there is general enthusiasm for making the change anyway, the cost is not particularly great, and the downside risks are no greater than the risks associated with making no change.
♦ Pick 90 percent if general enthusiasm is mild, the cost is middling, and the downside risks are not negligible.
♦ Pick 95 percent if general enthusiasm is lacking, the cost of the change is high, or if particular downside risks are appreciable.

TRIAL DURATION FOR CHANGES IN THE AVERAGE VALUE

The following procedure will produce the number of data points required to calculate the confidence interval about the average value, given a confidence level and a precision of result expressed in terms of the sample standard deviation.

Pick a confidence level, say 90 percent. Calculate the *significance level*, which is defined as one minus the confidence level; the significance level would be 10 percent, because the confidence level is 90 percent.

Make a rough guess of the number of data points, say 10. Then apply the Excel function T.INV(2 × SIGNIFICANCE LEVEL, 10). (The built-in function T.INV[. . .] returns the two-tailed answer, whereas the one-tailed answer is sought. To force this to work, double the significance level. This probably sounds backward, but it is so.) For a significance level of 10 percent and a count estimate of 10, the function reads T.INV(2 × 10%, 10) and returns 1.37.

One more parameter needs to be specified by the analyst: the precision of the outcome desired by the analyst expressed as a fraction of the sample standard deviation. One-quarter of a standard deviation is a possibility, or one-half. Pick, say, one-quarter of a standard deviation. With that selection in hand, calculate the number of data points by dividing the T.INV(. . .) result by the selected precision. In this case, that would be 1.37/0.25 = 5.49. Square this number; the square is an estimate of the number of data points required, in this case 30.13. Round that off to 30.

To confirm that the T.INV(. . .) function does not depend very much on the number of samples supplied as an argument, the T.INV(. . .) calculation can be repeated using 30 as the number of samples. Repeating the steps gives a T.INV value of 1.31 and a calculated number of data points equal to 27.48, so the number of data samples hardly changes. This is only a planning estimate, and an estimate of 27 is hardly different from an estimate of 30.

Here is that same example worked step by step:

Estimating Average Value Trial Length	
Confidence level	90%
Significance level	10%
Rough guess at number of data samples required	10
t-inverse value T.INV(2 × significance, rough guess)	1.37
Desired precision, fraction of sample standard deviation	0.25
That desired precision divided by the t-inverse value, in this case 0.25/1.37	5.49
That value squared	30.13
New sample count estimate, which is the previous value rounded off	30
Optional second iteration, replacing the rough guess with this new estimate	—
t-inverse value T.INV(2 × significance, new estimate)	1.31
Precision divided by this t-inverse value, squared	27.48
Improved estimate of sample size (the above), rounded	27

This is a good enough estimate for trial planning purposes.

Note that a fairly modest number of data samples is required to support a high-confidence outcome; this is because average values are very well behaved. The next table covers a reasonable range of confidence levels and precision. Recall that precision is defined in standard deviation units, so a precision of 0.50 means the sample average is within half a standard deviation of the true average.

Sample Size Required in Relation to Average Value			
Confidence level	75%	90%	95%
Significance level	25%	10%	5%
Precision in Standard Deviation Units			
1.00	3	4	5
0.50	3	8	13
0.25	8	27	45
0.10	46	166	272

Using this table and taking the same parameters used in the previous table, in which the confidence level is 90 percent and the precision is 0.25 standard deviations, we determine the required sample size is 27, which agrees with the prior analysis.

SAMPLE SIZE FOR THE STANDARD DEVIATION

If the purpose of the trial is to reduce the variability of a process, the trial needs to be run long enough to get a reasonable estimate of the new standard deviation. The development of a suitable sample size to estimate the distribution's standard deviation parallels the process used earlier to estimate the trial size when the average value is the primary interest, except that the chi-square distribution is used. The arithmetic is tedious, so it has been relegated to the website that accompanies this book, ache.org/books/6Sigma. The resulting table of multipliers is given here in tabular form and covers the likely range of interest.

Sample Size Required in Relation to Standard Deviation			
Confidence level	75%	90%	95%
Significance level	25%	10%	5%
Precision in Standard Deviation Units			
1.00	6	9	12
0.50	13	27	37
0.25	45	90	125
0.10	275	500	750

To apply this principle, select a confidence level and a precision and then read the number of samples required. For example, if a confidence level of 90 percent and a precision of 25 percent of the sample standard deviation are selected, read 90 as the number of samples required.

It will be observed that, for the same confidence level and the same precision, more samples are required to determine the standard deviation than to determine the average value. Furthermore, to achieve a higher precision in the standard deviation requires many, many more samples.

The analyst is required to select a precision before looking up the sample count in the table. The precision is a multiplier of the standard deviation of the sample. However, at this point, the standard deviation of the future sample is not known. Even so, the precision method is reasonable. When the trials are run and the samples are collected, some uncertainty will remain in the answers, and that uncertainty will be related to the standard deviation of the sample.

TESTING WITH VERY LOW ERROR RATES

Suppose we are tracking discrete events, some of which are errors. Let us further suppose that the error rate is very low. In testing processes with very low error rates, the trial may run for quite a long time without finding any errors. If the old process had a low error rate, too, figuring out whether the new system is any better than the old one might be difficult. Suppose the error rate in the old process is 1 per 1,000 events. If the process handles 2,000 events per month, gathering a sample set that includes several errors will take a long time. If the new process being put through the trial is expected to have 1 error per 1,000,000 events, the time spent completing the trial gets out of hand.

In the short run (during the trial), the question is whether the new system is in fact better than the old one. To answer this, a different distribution function will be brought to bear. An event that can have only one of two outcomes is called a *binomial event*. A binomial event has a probability of success and a probability of failure, and the sum of the two probabilities is unity.

Flip a coin. The probability of success in flipping heads is 50 percent, and the probability of *failing* to flip heads is 100 percent minus 50 percent, which equals 50 percent. Flip two coins at one time. The probability of success in flipping two heads is 25 percent, the probability of failing to flip two heads is 75 percent, and so on. Given a hat holding one red marble and two blue marbles, the probability of success in picking the red marble is 33.3 percent, and the probability of failure is 66.7 percent. What is the probability of flipping heads at least twice before flipping tails twice? Or of choosing the red marble twice before choosing one of the blue marbles?

Suppose the old system has a probability of success of 99.9 percent, which means that, on average, one error appears once in 1,000 cases. What is the likelihood of having 1,000 successes, 2,000 successes, or 3,000 successes before having *any* error?

Happily, a built-in spreadsheet function can perform this calculation; it is called the *negative binomial distribution.* In Excel, the function is NEGBINOMDIST(number of preceding failures, number of successes, probability of success). The function returns the probability that exactly that number of failures will transpire before exactly that number of successes, given the probability of success.

Applying this function and specifying no failures and 3,000 successes calls for the spreadsheet formula to be NEGBINOMDIST(0, 3000, 99.9%), which returns 4.97 percent; we will call it 5 percent. If 5 percent is the probability of having *no* errors in the first 3,000 tries, the probability of having *at least one error* must be 95 percent. To fill out the picture, here are a few more points:

Number of Tries Before Any Failure (Success Rate 99.9%)	
Tries	Probability
1,000	36.8%
2,000	13.5%
3,000	5.0%
4,000	1.8%
5,000	0.7%
10,000	< 0.1%

To summarize the table, the old system could be expected to have zero-error runs of 1,000 tries 37 percent of the time, zero-error runs of 3,000 tries only 5 percent of the time, and zero-error runs of 5,000 tries less than 1 percent of the time.

So, if the goal is to run the trial long enough to be 95 percent confident that the new system is better than the old one, the trial must be run long enough that the old system would be 95 percent likely to produce an error, which is about 3,000 tries. If the confidence level requirement is raised to 99 percent, the trial needs to run through about 5,000 tries. By that time, the old system would have, with 99 percent confidence, produced at least one error. If the new system produces no errors in that time, the new system is, with 99 percent confidence, better than the old one. How much better? The same NEGBINOMDIST(. . .) function can be applied on a trial-and-error basis to find out what the error rate for the new process can be if the trial produces zero errors in the first run of 2,000 samples. Doing so gives the result that, with 75 percent confidence, the error rate for the new process is not higher than 144 per million events. If the first 5,000 samples include no errors, the new process's error rate, with 75 percent confidence, is not higher than 60 per million events.

TESTING THE HYPOTHESIS

Test the hypothesis by running the trial long enough to generate a sufficient number of samples, and analyze the results. The standard statistical tests that are available are the t-test for the average value and the F-test for the standard deviation. These answer the questions, "Is the average still the same after the process change, and with what confidence?" and "Is the standard deviation still the same after the process change, and with what confidence?" With a spreadsheet such as Excel, these tests are easy to apply. However, both are rather conservative and may be frustrating in real applications.

What is more rewarding is to track progress with control charts. Although the eye may be fooled by distributions that are nearly the same, the eye is not likely to be fooled if a significant change is seen between the old process and the new one.

Exhibit 9.3: Tracking Chart—The Trial Begins

If the improvement is so small that the eye is fooled, there is no point in studying this candidate change any further.

In the control chart shown in exhibit 9.3, some of the data from the old system are included for reference, and the old process control limits and system limits are shown. The start of the trial is marked, and the new data are plotted to the right of this event, using filled circles. In this case, the data are clearly clustering at a lower point on the page and, so far, seem to be more closely bunched.

When 20 or so new data points are available, new control charts can be generated with new control limits and new system limits. The spreadsheet functions T.TEST(. . .) and F.TEST(. . .) can be applied to complement the visual inspection of progress.

FACTORIAL EXPERIMENTS

A factorial experimental series is one in which two or more changes are considered in various combinations. In a factory, various machine setting combinations can be tried and the best ones selected for production.

In a healthcare organization, setting up combinatorial testing is practically impossible; it is too complicated, and it takes too long. Other outside influences are likely to fog the data. In actuality, the issue is rather the reverse, as healthcare always involves variable factors that cannot be eliminated. For example, if the health service runs 24 hours a day, the selection of which shift is studied might affect the outcome of the trial; so might weekend versus weekday; so might variation in patient care unit. Just listing these built-in combinations gives us something approaching a factorial experiment.

There is a simple way to organize these combinations and to extract some information from them, particularly identifying those variables that seem to have a large influence on the results. This information may make it possible to isolate the key variables for further study.

Here is another example. A hospital wants to know if adding more paraprofessional staff to the patient care units will decrease the time it takes to deliver the mid-shift medication to each patient. One would hope so, but a Scottish dictum tells us, "One boy is a boy, two boys are less than a boy, and three boys are no boy at all." The three patient care units and four shifts during the week provide a lot of variables to ponder. Also, the hospital wonders if striking a gong at the mid-shift hour would get the medication round started on time and, perhaps, ended on time. Data are gathered, with the following outcomes:

Gong	Paras.	Shift 1	Shift 2	Shift 3	Time
−1	1	1	−1	−1	34.0
−1	2	1	−1	−1	27.0
−1	3	1	−1	−1	23.0
−1	1	−1	1	−1	27.0
−1	2	−1	1	−1	25.0
−1	3	−1	1	−1	23.0
−1	1	−1	−1	1	21.0
−1	2	−1	−1	1	20.0
−1	3	−1	−1	1	19.0
−1	1	−1	−1	−1	41.0
−1	2	−1	−1	−1	38.0
−1	3	−1	−1	−1	33.0
1	1	1	−1	−1	17.0
1	2	1	−1	−1	13.5
1	3	1	−1	−1	11.5
1	1	−1	1	−1	13.5
1	2	−1	1	−1	12.5
1	3	−1	1	−1	11.5
1	1	−1	−1	1	10.5
1	2	−1	−1	1	10.0
1	3	−1	−1	1	9.5
1	1	−1	−1	−1	20.5
1	2	−1	−1	−1	19.0
1	3	−1	−1	−1	16.5

The heading "Paras" is the number of paraprofessionals on the patient care unit. The entries under "Gong" and the different shifts are numeric values implying "no" and "yes" to whether the gong was struck; any numeric values would do here. For the shifts, if Shift 1 is true, then Shifts 2 and 3 are false, and so on. The "Time" heading indicates the number of minutes taken to dispense the medication.

With numeric values in every square, regression analysis takes over. Using spreadsheet regression and identifying time as the y-value and the five other columns as x-values, the regression tool creates the relationship between variables and outcomes. The fitted equation has a coefficient for each of the variables, and every coefficient is accompanied by a confidence interval.

As has now been shown many times in this book, if only a few sample data points are available, the confidence intervals are so wide as to be useless. Take that as a true message: There is a great uncertainty in the fitted values. Let us put the fitted coefficients aside and look at another output from the analysis.

In Excel, if the box LINE-FIT CHARTS is checked on the REGRESSION panel, the program will produce several simple charts, each of which shows the given data points and the fitted points. Exhibit 9.4 shows the chart for the gong variable. Dependence on the gong variable is shown by the data points on the left (no gong) being substantially higher on the page than the points on the right (yes gong). Looking at the other plots, which can be found on the website that accompanies this book, ache.org/books/6Sigma, one sees much less dependence on those other variables.

Exhibit 9.4: Gong Line-Fit Plot

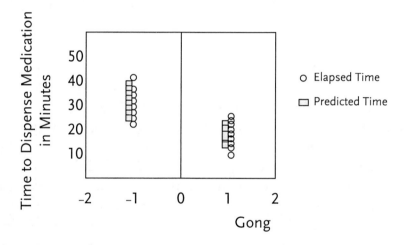

Thus the regression analysis provides the service of organizing these simple data charts, which facilitate sorting the important variables from the less important variables. A statistician may be able to glean the same information from the many statistical characteristics provided by the analysis, but there is nothing in those numbers that is not obvious to the eye in these charts.

Note that there is no requirement that every combination be covered in the table; what is required is that a numeric value be given in each case to represent true or false, as was done with the gong variable above. If some squares are blank, leave out those rows. It is up to the reader to decide whether the idea that a gong gets everybody moving constitutes useful management guidance.

AN INTEGRATED EXAMPLE

The following scenario serves as an integrated example. Note that it does not reflect any real experience, nor does it imply in any way that such events could happen in any healthcare organization. This example is simply offered because it shows the Six Sigma approach to analyzing important situations and can be understood by the lay reader.

The Event

A staff nurse prepares to inject a patient with a prescribed drug. Then the nurse makes a new calculation of the correct dosage of the drug, considering the patient's age and weight. Upon completing and rechecking the new calculation, the nurse decides the prescribed dosage is much too great, stops the injection, and notifies management and the attending physician through established channels.

The Standing Procedure

Although many medications come in "adult" and "child" sizes, others are prescribed in proportion to the patient's body weight, typically in milligrams per kilogram. The heart drug Digoxin and some other medications are prescribed in milligrams for adults and micrograms per kilogram of body weight for infants.

A physician prescribes the medication. If the medication is prescribed according to body weight, the physician uses the body weight from the patient's record, does the arithmetic, and decides on the quantity of medicine for that patient. If the physician prescribes this particular medicine frequently, the unit quantities are immediately available to the physician by rote; if this physician prescribes this particular medicine infrequently, a reference book is consulted for the quantities. A charge nurse notes the prescribed dose and duplicates the calculations. If there is agreement between the physician's and nurse's calculations, the order is sent to the pharmacy.

The pharmacist receives the order, checks the prescribed medicine against the patient's known allergies and against other medication this patient is known to be taking, and checks the dosage against the patient's body weight. The patient information is taken from the patient's record. If no conflict is found, the pharmacist fills the order and sends it to the patient care unit.

A staff nurse in the patient care unit checks the delivery from the pharmacy against the physician's original prescription and delivers the medicine to the patient.

The staff nurse also considers whether the dose seems to be consistent with the patient's body weight, making a new calculation if in doubt.

Action

Hospital management assigns a project sponsor from the senior management ranks. The sponsoring senior manager selects a Six Sigma black belt to lead the project. The project leader meets with the line managers from the concerned departments and conveys management's directive that the issue be resolved and management's request that all parties provide full cooperation and support. The sponsoring senior manager confirms that this is management's position, giving each person present a firm look in the eye.

The project leader asks if anyone remembers other similar cases in the past year or so. Two or three people mention cases that, although they were not exactly the same, they remember being in the same ballpark. The group concludes that this case cannot be declared unique. The group also agrees that the same might recur at any time and, because of this, that some stop-gap mechanism should be applied immediately. The group performs a fishbone analysis to identify likely causes and to make sure the entire group has a common understanding of the issues.

The group agrees that the hospital records should be examined for comparable events. The patient care staff should be encouraged to recollect comparable events. Procedures from comparable hospitals should be examined to provide a benchmark against which the present process as well as any candidate for a future process can be tested.

Stop-Gap Measures

Given the serious nature of the issue, the group considers that some stop-gap measures need to be put in place and applied until a full analysis can be completed. The stop-gap measures will break the chain of events. The group recognizes that any stop-gap measure will add to operating expense and may well slow down the normal processing times. Given the gravity of the issue, the group considers that management will support the stop-gap measures.

The group considers what measures to apply. After some discussion, the group settles on inserting one additional check of the medication order at the patient care unit, after the pharmacy order is delivered to the patient care unit and before the medicine delivery round is started. This check will be done by a registered nurse, and the check will be included in the patient's record as well as in a project log.

Exhibit 9.5: Extra-Check Potential Problem Analysis

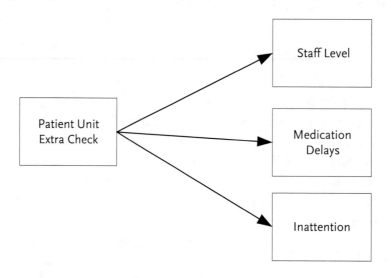

The group considers the potential problems with this measure, which are captured in the management-level chart shown in exhibit 9.5.

The recognized potential problems are as follows:

1. The extra workload on the staff nurses needs to be considered, and it may be necessary to add a nurse per patient care unit during this stop-gap period.
2. The time taken to do the extra checking after the pharmacy order is delivered means that there will be some additional delay before the round can begin. Because it may take half an hour to do the checking, the delay can bunch work up and interfere with other duties.
3. The routine nature of this overchecking may become so mechanical that the person doing the overchecking does not give full attention to the task, thereby following the bathtub failure model.

After some discussion, the group revises the plan to take care of these potential problems:

1. The overcheck will not be done after the pharmacy order is delivered; rather, the overcheck will be done between the time the physician gives the order and the time the pharmacy delivers the order, working from the pharmacy order and the patient's record. This will not catch errors made in the pharmacy, but the group considers these the least likely. The group judges that one or two nurses per shift can do the overchecking for all patient care

units, moving from unit to unit. The patient care unit head nurse will do the overchecking for those exceptional cases where time so requires.

2. A senior nursing supervisor will spot-check the overchecks on a sample basis to keep the attention level high.

3. The staff nurse, before delivering the medication, will check both the original physician's order and the overcheck entry in the patient's record.

4. All errors of any kind will be reported to the project office so a data record can be accumulated.

5. The overcheck nurses will report on their experience to the project office and provide timely reports to line management.

6. The project leader will walk the floors from time to time to gather anecdotal input from patient care unit personnel, pharmacy personnel, physicians, and others—indeed, information will be collected from anyone who has anything to say.

Gathering the Data

Patient records are studied for the prior 20 months, which is the longest period of time for which the records are reasonably available. This study shows that the error rate is about 1 per 1,000 when all manner of similar errors are considered. Few if any of these errors were actually life-threatening, but the point of the study is to gather information about how the system works.

The data are as follows:

Month	Error Rate per 1,000	Month	Error Rate per 1,000
June	2.1	May	1.1
July	0.4	June	0.3
August	0.6	July	1.3
September	1.7	August	1.5
October	0.4	September	1.3
November	0.5	October	1.2
December	0	November	0.5
January	1.0	December	1.2
February	0.2	January	0.7
March	1.4	**Average**	**1.0**
April	2.1	**Standard Deviation**	**0.8**

From these data, the analyst calculates Six Sigma system limits at zero on the lower side and average-plus-six-times-the-standard-deviation on the upper side, which is to say 5.8 errors per 1,000. The process control limits, which are three standard deviations away from the average value, are at zero and 3.4 errors per 1,000.

The analyst considers subgroups of data and finds no appreciable dependence on shift, patient care unit, patient age category, use of a common drug versus an uncommon drug, or any other parameter anyone in the group could imagine. The error rate is low in all cases, so the sample size in the subgroups is too low to provide much guidance.

Assessing the Stop-Gap Measures

The project leader calls a meeting of the group. The analyst presents the information and the system limits. Upon discussion, the group decides the previously prescribed stop-gap measures will cover the range from zero to 6 errors per 1,000. The group and the leader make the following recommendations to management:

1. The stop-gap measures should be continued until further notice.
2. Any concomitant changes in staffing, work scheduling, or standard costs should be made permanent.
3. Data gathering should continue.
4. Work should be done to identify a system weakness; the group believes this weakness exists, as the problem cannot be localized.
5. Consideration should be given to changes in the system that would provide a substantial reduction in the error rate.

Implications of the Six Sigma System Limits

With the stop-gap measures in place, the group believes the error rate will be much lower than the previous 1 per thousand, although not yet enough data are in hand to say that the error rate will be as low as 3.4 per million. Performance will be tracked and, as data are accumulated, the error rate will be quantified.

The stop-gap efforts add extra nursing effort and therefore add to operating costs. The stop-gap efforts, by allowing time for a replacement pharmacy order if necessary, dilate the time required to complete the pharmacy order process. Both of these are negatives.

This issue can be considered in two parts. The added nursing effort is internal to the process; it now costs more to execute this process. The time dilation is external to the process and affects the overall system. Other parties need to adjust their schedules to accommodate the time dilation. A change in system limits always affects other parties.

The group believes that the added cost and the changed system limits, even with their effects on other parties, are the correct management action to take in the short run because the pharmacy order error rate will be brought down substantially. The group asks management to accept the cost and asks the other parties to accept the changed system limits.

The group now pursues improvement of the cost and the system limits by seeking other sufficient solutions. This means the group will only consider changes to the process that will have error rates on the order of 3.4 per million and that it will not consider changes that save money and time but that do not reduce the error rate to approximately 3.4 per million.

Failure Modes and Effects Analysis

The pre-existing system had four checks in series: the physician checked his or her own work, the attending nurse calculated the dosage independently, the pharmacist calculated the dosage independently, and the patient care unit nurse checked the delivered medication against the original order and against common practice. For the wrong dosage to reach the patient, four independent failures had to happen.

Failure mode and effects charts (exhibit 9.6), prepared by an analyst working with nurses, pharmacists, and physicians from the project group, help visualize the process, identify weak spots, and find common sources of error.

Exhibit 9.6: Dosage Failure Mode Analysis

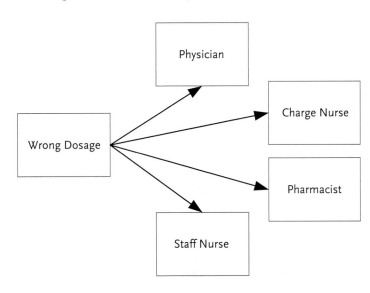

For each of the actors, an additional failure mode and effects chart was produced by the same group (exhibits 9.7 and 9.8). The charts for the charge nurse and the pharmacist looked the same, so only one is included here.

Exhibit 9.7: Failure Mode Chart for the Physician

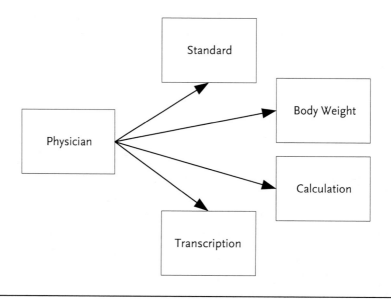

Exhibit 9.8: Failure Mode Chart for the Charge Nurse

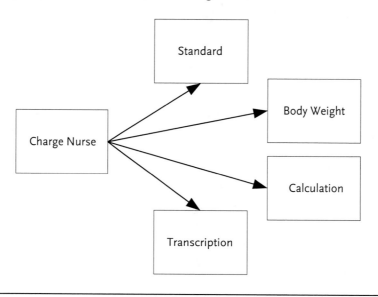

The chart for the patient care unit staff nurse (exhibit 9.9) is a little different:

Exhibit 9.9: Failure Mode Chart for the Staff Nurse

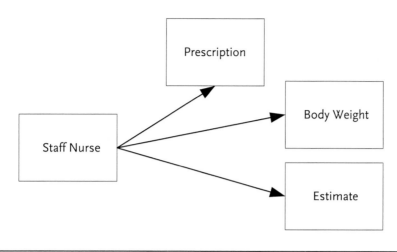

The four charts clearly indicate that there is one candidate for common-mode error: the body weight (exhibit 9.10).

Exhibit 9.10: Common Failure Mode Analysis

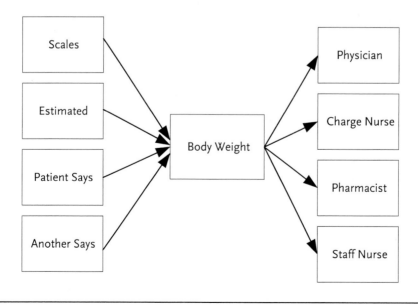

Further investigation reveals that the hospital routinely weighs infants and small children, and there is no reason to believe the scales are unreliable. Ambulatory adults are weighed, but nonambulatory patients may or may not be weighed. If the adult patient is not weighed, the staff either make an estimate based on experience or ask the patient or an accompanying family member for the estimated weight. The group believes the estimates are probably accurate within 20 percent, that the patient is probably accurate within 20 percent, and that the weight guessed by an accompanying family member is very imprecise.

The data show that in at least one case of interest, the patient was a small child who had been weighed at the hospital on standard scales. So, although this is a weak spot in the system, it cannot be the only one.

No other common sources of error connect to all four actors, but there is one that connects the physician and the attending nurse: the calculation and transcription act. Although the charge nurse is trained to provide an independent calculation and transcription, anecdotal information tells the group that the nurses are subject to distraction and that they are more likely to believe the doctor's calculations than their own. In other words, the independent check is not completely independent.

The pharmacist is completely independent in that he or she performs separate calculations away from the bedside. Indeed, some of the included cases in the database are errors caught by the pharmacist. The patient care unit staff nurse does not perform a calculation but relies only on experience and training to recognize unusual cases. The staff nurse does, however, check the pharmacy order against the pharmacy delivery.

Three-Plane Modeling

The group elected to consider the three-plane portrayal of the situation to see if any conditions or constraints need further attention. The main elements, in the group's opinion, are shown in the following table:

| Three-Plane Model of the Pharmacy Order Issue | | |
Mechanisms	Conditions	Constraints
Physician prescribes medicine	Patient's weight often estimated, not measured	Manual bedside system; pharmacist has computer cross-check facility
Charge nurse confirms	Charge nurses tend to discount their own calculations and accept the physician's	Policy is to weigh patients, but there is no way to do so for bedfast patients and some emergency patients

(continued)

(continued from previous page)

Mechanisms	Conditions	Constraints
Pharmacist checks	Pharmacist works from patient's record	Manual order-writing system; manual bedside cross-checking system
Staff nurse considers	Physician may make decimal error or call up wrong dose from memory	System is an open loop, with no feedback to the physician or charge nurse before drug is given to patient
Expectation	Staff nurse will catch gross errors on familiar drugs but probably not those on less-familiar drugs	No peer review of physician's prescription

The group finds the three-plane portrayal interesting because the constraints plane identifies those matters that management will wish to address in the longer term. Management cannot do much about the conditions but can change the constraints. The group takes note that the constraints plane has one new matter: peer review (or rather the lack of peer review) of the physician's prescription. The group decides, after discussing the matter, that this is too far afield, because the charge to the group is to deal with errors downstream of the diagnosis. This may be a suitable topic for separate consideration later or for research into computer-supported bedside diagnostic methods or other future technology.

Group's Conclusions

The group draws the following conclusions:

1. The hospital should weigh all patients who receive weight-dependent medication.
2. The hospital should provide independent bedside calculation and transcription of pharmacy orders.
3. Emphasis should be given to adding technology to address the conditions rather than to adding manual checking or other manual steps.

The group recommends that practices of comparable hospitals be reviewed, vendors be contacted, and suitable trials of candidate changes be undertaken. It also recommends continuing the data gathering and the stop-gap measures until further notice.

Management Action

Hospital management issues an order that all patients be weighed as part of the admitting process. For those patients who must be medicated before it is possible to weigh them, the hospital orders that caution be used in prescribing weight-dependent medication and that the patient be weighed at the first opportunity, with confirmation of any intervening medication dosage.

Hospital management authorizes the project leader to undertake trials to find better systems for precluding bedside calculation and transcription errors.

TRIAL OF A HANDHELD DEVICE

From various vendor offerings, the project leader, in consultation with the group, selects a handheld computer device with a small screen and wand. The handheld computer contains data on 400 medications, including information about standard dosage, adult dosage, infant dosage, weight-dependent dosage, and the like. The device does not have a printer, but it can send information to a personal computer at the patient care unit station at the end of the round. The device's wand is a bar-code reader that picks up the patient's barcode from his or her record. The wand also acts as a stylus, enabling the user to tap the device screen to select a medication, enter a body weight, and so on.

A question then arises: Should both the physician and the charge nurse have one of these devices, or should just the physician or just the nurse have one? After consulting with physicians and nurses, the project leader decides that, for the first trial, the charge nurse will be issued the handheld device rather than the physician. The physician will continue to make calculations in the traditional way.

Two patient care units are selected for the trial. A total of ten handheld devices are acquired. The vendor provides additional on-site support during the trial in the hope of winning an eventual order for more substantial quantities.

Trial Duration

The current error rate is 1 per 1,000 pharmacy orders. The hospital has 200 acute care beds plus an outpatient service, so the number of pharmacy orders is about 2,000 per month.

The analyst believes there is general support for a change such as the introduction of a handheld device because the hospital is evaluating electronic records and other data-automation concepts and the staff are generally interested in computer devices. The handheld devices are not burdensomely expensive. Therefore, the analyst believes the trial should be designed to a confidence level of 75 percent.

The trial should endure until the new average value is determined to a precision of about half a standard deviation. The "Number of Tries Before Any Failure" table on page 153 leads the analyst to conclude that about 3,000 samples of pharmacy orders will be required. At the current rate of 2,000 pharmacy orders per month, it would take about six weeks to get 3,000 samples if the whole hospital were involved in the trial. Upon inspection, it is decided that the two patient care units being tested generate about one-third of the total pharmacy orders, so to get a total of 3,000 pharmacy orders from these two patient care units will take about ten weeks.

The old system had some months with no errors. Because this is true, there is a reasonable likelihood that the two patient care units, using the old system, would have periods of ten weeks with no errors at all. Therefore, running with no errors for two or three months may or may not provide sufficient evidence that the new system is actually better than the old system; some analysis is required. Applying the negative binomial distribution to determine the likelihood that 3,000 successful outcomes will happen before the first error gives the likelihood of about 5 percent. So, under the old system, any 3,000 successive pharmacy orders will have at least one error, with a likelihood of 95 percent; the analyst can be 95 percent confident that, if no errors are found in the first 3,000 pharmacy orders during the trial, the new system is an improvement over the old system. This result is better than the 75 percent confidence level requirement set by the analyst, so it is accepted.

Thus, the trial evaluation method will be as follows:

1. Run the trial until the trial patient care units have issued 3,000 pharmacy orders, which will take about ten weeks.
2. Expect no errors during that time.
3. If even one error occurs during the trial, the new system cannot be shown to be better than the old system.

Trial Execution

Nurses were selected from among a group of volunteers, and general cooperation by the physicians was granted. The nurses were trained on the new device.

The nurses conducted a potential problem analysis, which involved considering the following: any ripple effects of carrying one more device on the rounds, the responsibility for transferring the patient data from the handheld device to the patient care unit computer at the end of the rounds, the responsibility to print out the patient data sheet and include it in the patient's record, and the question of whether the nurse's signature should be affixed to the printed form or if the nurse's name entered into the handheld device would be sufficient. Questions of battery replacement and what to do if the device gets lost or damaged were also aired.

The hospital's information technology department assigned one person to be the go-to contact for any problems with the handheld device. The vendor's on-site representative pledged to be available immediately, or at least promptly, in response to a page.

A pretrial period of three days was declared, during which the nurses would use the handheld device just to get the hang of it, with no entries going into patient records. This was intended to address the likely "infant mortality" errors as people got used to the new devices.

The trial ran for ten weeks. No errors were observed. Nurses found the handheld devices could be carried in a pocket without much bother. The data transfer at the end of the round was taken over by the patient care unit clerk. Nurses adopted the habit of checking the patient's record on the next round to be sure the calculation record was there. Physicians got in the habit of checking the handheld device for dose standards for drugs not commonly used, just to verify their recollection of the standards.

Nurses found they sometimes made an error, most commonly a decimal error, when entering the body weight into the handheld device, but as this calculation was completely independent of the physician's calculation, the discrepancy was immediately noted in every such event and corrected on the spot. This was not counted as an error because it did not increase the risk to the patient. Two handheld devices were lost or damaged during the trial. These were replaced from the inventory of spares.

In walking the floors to talk to the people involved, the Six Sigma project leader received 27 suggestions for other features the handheld device might incorporate to make it more useful to the users. These were logged for future evaluation.

Long-Term Tracking

Tracking of the pharmacy order error rate continues over the long term to make sure that the process does not degrade over time. A periodic report is created that flows to the affected parties and to management.

Cost–Benefit Analysis

The cost–benefit analysis compares two sufficient solutions: the stop-gap solution and the new-technology solution. The lease cost for the handheld devices is found to be less than $5 per day per patient care unit. The stop-gap cost of the extra nursing effort is found to be $50 per day per patient care unit. On the basis of cost alone, the new-technology solution is preferred.

The time dilation, which is represented by the system limits that go with the stop-gap measures, is not easily expressed in dollar terms. Therefore, the comparison between the stop-gap and the new-technology solutions has to be expressed in nonmonetary terms. The new-technology solution allows the system limits to be revised to reflect the removal of the time dilation, which is favorable. Therefore, the cost analysis and the improvements in the system limits both favor the new-technology solution.

There would be no point in attempting to apply a cost–benefit analysis to a change from the old process to any new process because the old process (without the stop-gap measures) was unacceptable, no matter how favorable its costs. Cost–benefit analysis is appropriate only when comparing sufficient solutions.

Conclusion of the Event

At the end of the trial period, the project leader met with the group once again. Upon discussion of the information received, the group made the following recommendations:

1. The handheld device trial should be considered a success and be extended to the balance of the hospital in an orderly progression, with due consideration given to special circumstances, such as emergency department service.
2. Data logging should be continued, and periodic reports should be issued to management and to interested parties.
3. The patient care unit level overchecking should be discontinued, as the handheld device use will now extend to the whole hospital. The nurses doing the overchecking work should be reassigned.
4. The several suggestions for added functionality should be circulated for consideration by interested parties, with no commitment at this stage.
5. Although the body-weight estimation issue seems to have caused no errors during the trial period, further consideration should be given to finding ways to weigh bedfast or otherwise hard-to-weigh adult and adolescent

patients. Responsibility for this matter should be assigned to an appropriate senior staff member for resolution.

6. The project report should now be filed and the project case closed.
7. Senior management should express its thanks to the many people who participated in making the trial a success.

Six Sigma Conclusion

Performance of the system is what counts.

To GET THE system to work well, it is necessary to get the employees to work well and to get management to manage well. Employees work well when the tasks they perform are designed under the poka-yoke guidelines and the work flows in a sensible way. Management manages well when facts are organized and information is quantified, when problems get solved, when new problems are detected before they become serious, and when change is managed. Both management and employees respond to worthy goals.

Six Sigma—by setting the worthy goal of 3.4 errors per million opportunities; applying poka-yoke guidelines to the design of work tasks; reducing variability; providing systematic problem-solving and problem-detecting methods; and providing a systematic, quantitative method for managing change—is a worthwhile management method with useful applicability to healthcare.

Remember, it's never the person, it's always the system when something goes awry.

The aim of the High-Reliability Organization is to inculcate a culture that anticipates and corrects—a culture that includes employees, professionals, and management. Six Sigma supports the High-Reliability Organization.

Cases will follow in the next chapters. Working the cases is good. Simply reading the cases is good, too. New information has been added to every case. The companion website (ache.org/books/6Sigma) provides an Excel workbook that includes a worksheet for every case, with the data already entered.

Cases

The following cases are provided for those readers who wish to apply the lessons of the book. In particular, readers following a Six Sigma training program with a Six Sigma trainer to achieve green belt or black belt certification will find the cases are organized to help them achieve their goals.

The cases introduce additional material to extend mastery beyond what has been provided in the text of the book. For those who wish to delve even deeper into workflow analysis, bonus cases serve as mental exercises.

CASE OVERVIEW

These are practical cases that provide practice in computer modeling of a situation using a spreadsheet—what some would call evidence-driven analysis. The first ten cases are basic analysis suitable for a Six Sigma green belt training program. Cases in the second series are more advanced, and are suitable for a Six Sigma black belt training program.

The Green Belt Series of Cases

Six Sigma green belt certification asserts that the certified green belt holder is competent to carry out Six Sigma projects. The first ten cases apply Six Sigma principles. The trainer for a green belt class may wish to assign these first ten cases. The trainer may also assign a special project to each student, or, for variety, substitute other cases that cover the same material.

Many of these cases include data sets. The sets are provided in Excel format on the companion website, ache.org/books/6Sigma, to save the student tedious typing.

The Black Belt Series of Cases

Six Sigma black belt certification asserts that the certified black belt holder is competent to design Six Sigma projects and to supervise their execution. The trainer for a black belt class may wish to assign the green belt series and, in addition, cases 11 through 20. The trainer will also assign a special project to each student that will include the design and execution of a trial. For variety, the trainer may substitute other cases that cover the same material.

The Bonus Series of Cases

The bonus series does not require much arithmetic, but the cases do require some thought. The lessons taught in the book may guide the thinking to good effect.

Spreadsheet Use

These cases require a spreadsheet computer application such as Microsoft Excel 2016. Those who do not have prior experience using a spreadsheet would benefit from doing a tutorial series before starting these cases. Tutorials are commonly provided with the application and may be found by selecting the help menu and searching for "tutorial." If no tutorial is readily at hand, please look into the "icebreaker" Excel file on this book's companion website. The icebreaker exercises cover all the fundamental spreadsheet operations that are required to complete the cases. As with most computer applications, asking questions of a more experienced user is productive; although the operations are simple enough once they are known, they are baffling to the first-time user.

THE COMPANION WEBSITE

The companion website, ache.org/books/6Sigma, includes the following:

1. An Excel template containing all the case input data for each case
2. An Excel file providing additional details on the examples used in the text and the appendixes

3. PowerPoint presentation templates
4. Two completed case reports for general guidance
5. An icebreaker spreadsheet

The Excel files are in "template" format. The user can load these files, make entries, and save the resulting file as an Excel spreadsheet model. The template file remains pristine and can be used again *de novo*. A trainer may wish to make various modifications and additions to these templates and save the result as a new template file, using the "save as" function.

CASE 1: DATA PORTRAYAL

Drill on Applying Six Sigma

Cases 1, 2, and 3 are a set. In these cases, basic Six Sigma data portrayal and analysis are applied to the data sets provided. The standard spreadsheet tools are applied.

Topic: Tool Drill

These days, most personal computers have a sufficient set of tools to facilitate the data analysis and portrayal that are necessary parts of Six Sigma projects. This first case applies those tools to the set of data provided in the next section. The data set also is provided in digital form on the companion website, ache.org /books/6Sigma.

Students who have no prior experience using a spreadsheet computer application would do well to run through a tutorial. If no tutorial is readily available, the novice may wish to work through the icebreaker Excel sheet on the website that accompanies this book, which walks through the fundamentals. Because this icebreaker is limited in scope, working through a full tutorial at the first opportunity is a good idea.

A complete solution to this case also is provided on the companion website.

Work

1. Calculate the average and the standard deviation for the data set using the built-in functions AVERAGE(. . .) and STDEV.P(. . .).

2. Calculate the process control limits, which are defined as three standard deviations above and below the average. Make two new columns on the spreadsheet and copy these limits into those columns so that one column is all upper process control limit and the other is all lower control limit. These will be used for plotting. These cells will have one column for the upper limit, the cells of which have the same value, and one column for the lower limit, the cells of which have the same value.

3. Calculate the system limits, which are at six standard deviations above and below the average. If the lower limit dips below zero, use zero as the lower limit. Make a column on the spreadsheet for the lower system limit and the upper system limit, as above. The upper limit cells will all have the same value. The lower limit cells will all have the same value.

4. Plot a scatter diagram, which is made up of points not connected by lines. To do this, select all the data columns, including the counter column. From the INSERT menu, select CHART, then choose the SCATTER DIAGRAM option, and follow the rest of the instructions. Include the data, the process control limits, and the system limits, which will all show up as dots. Finish this chart.

5. Using the completed chart, change the upper process control limit to a line. To do this, right-click on one of the upper process control limit points on the graph to get a pop-up menu. Select FORMAT DATA SERIES. In the left panel titled LINE, select AUTOMATIC. In the right panel titled MARKER, select NONE. Close the menu. Repeat this process for the other limit lines.

6. Save the spreadsheet with a suitable name.

Now, let's create a histogram of the data.

1. From the TOOLS menu, select DATA ANALYSIS, and then HISTOGRAM. If the TOOLS menu does not show DATA ANALYSIS on its list, it is necessary to activate DATA ANALYSIS before it can be used. This is easy to do. Start again; select TOOLS, then ADD-INS, and then ANALYSIS TOOLPAK. Close this menu. Select the TOOLS menu again; now, the DATA ANALYSIS option will appear at the bottom of the list.

2. The HISTOGRAM tool requires that the user identify the bins that the tool will drop the data into. Create a column of bins starting at zero and running to 3.0 in increments of 0.1. The first few entries will be 0, 0.1, 0.2, 0.3, and so on. Run the HISTOGRAM tool.

   Caution: The tool does not run itself again every time the sheet is recalculated the way a built-in function does. Therefore, the analyst must rerun the HISTOGRAM tool if the data change.

3. Run the HISTOGRAM tool again. The panel will show the same entries, so this part will be quick. Check the plot option, run the tool, and then close the box. Edit the plot a little by changing the title, deleting the legend, and tweaking other elements as desired. To make these updates, click on the item of interest to get a pop-up menu, then experiment. If you do not like what you see, use the UNDO feature in the EDIT menu to back up.

Data

Use this data set; it can also be found on the companion website, ache.org /books/6Sigma.

1.74	1.29	1.55	1.58	1.49
1.37	1.78	1.20	1.53	1.40
1.70	1.34	1.45	1.49	1.22
1.40	1.30	1.31	1.54	1.36
1.56	1.75	1.39	2.10	1.39
1.44	1.50	1.47	1.26	1.33

Analysis

If the process is undergoing normal fluctuations, 99.7 percent of the observations will fall within the process control limit band, by definition of the normal distribution. So, any point that falls outside the process control limits is a point to be studied further. It is not necessarily true that that point is wrong or that the process has suddenly gone out of control; rather, the point is so unusual that it invites close scrutiny.

Points that fall outside the system limits occur only a few times in a million, so any point falling there is a cause for alarm. Something is wrong; sound the claxon.

In the case report, remark on any points that fall outside the band. Mark any such points with an arrow or another highlight on the scatter diagram and on the histogram. If no points fall outside of the bands, remark to this effect in the report. To put a halo around a point on the chart, select the chart, go to the VIEW menu, and select TOOLBARS, which causes a submenu to appear. Select DRAWING. Drawing tools will appear across the bottom of the Excel screen. Select the OVAL tool. Drag the mouse across the target data point and unclick. An oval will be drawn over the data point. The oval will probably be filled, which obscures the data point. To eliminate the fill, select the oval, right-click to get the PROPERTIES menu, then select FORMAT AUTOSHAPE. Select the tab called COLORS AND LINES. Under the FILL section of the panel, drop down the list next to COLOR. At the top of the list is NO FILL; select this. Close the menu. The oval will now be a halo around the data point. Repeat the formatting process to set the oval's line to a suitable color. On the chart, select and drag the oval to position it suitably around the target data point.

Lessons Learned

You have now applied the basic tools, created a control chart with limits, observed aberrant points, and created a report for management.

CASE 2: PROCESS TRACKING

Topic: Process Observation and Analysis

The process control diagram created in case 1 will be retained, and new data will be plotted on the same diagram. The new data will be observed to fall—or not fall—within the bands. Additional analysis will test the change in average value and standard deviation.

Work

1. Use the new data set in the next section. Use the same process control limits and system limits that were found in case 1. Create a scatter diagram.
2. Observe that this data set seems to be off a little from the center of the bands. To see if this is within normal fluctuations, calculate confidence intervals for the new and old data sets.
3. Calculate the average and the standard deviation for the new data set. In addition, select a confidence level of 90 percent. Calculate the significance level by subtracting the confidence level from unity to get—in this case, 10 percent.
   Average value confidence interval: To calculate the confidence interval for the average value, calculate the Student's t-factor for this data set, which has 30 data samples, by using the built-in function T.INV(twice the significance factor, number of samples)—in this case T.INV(20%, 30). Multiply this by the standard deviation of the new data set. Add and subtract this from the set average value to get the confidence limits on the average value.

4. Repeat the previous step using the average and standard deviation from case 1. Compare the results.

5. Think of some way to plot the confidence intervals so that they can be compared directly by observation.

6. *Standard deviation confidence interval*: To set the confidence interval on the standard deviation with the same confidence factor and significance factor, calculate two factors using the chi-square distribution built-in functions.

    Lower multiplier: Calculate CHIINV[(significance level/2), sample count less one]. Using 90 percent confidence and 30 samples, that will be CHIINV(5%, 29). Divide the result into the sample-count-less-one, which in this case is 29. Take the square root of the result using SQRT(. . .); this gives the lower multiplier. Multiply the sample standard deviation by this result to get the lower confidence limit on the standard deviation.

    Upper multiplier: Repeat this process for the upper limit, this time using CHIINV[(1 − significance level/2), sample count less one] or, in this case, CHIINV(95%, 29).

7. One way to compare samples is to compare the confidence intervals on their average values and standard deviations. Repeat the previous step using the standard deviation for the data set from case 1. Because the data sets are the same size, the multipliers are in fact the same.

8. Think of some way to plot the two sets of confidence intervals so that they can be compared directly by observation. Take care to distinguish the confidence intervals of the average from the confidence intervals of the standard deviation.

9. Note for future reference that the previous procedure can be generalized by using the built-in function COUNT(. . .) to get the size of the sample set.

10. Include the scatter diagram and the confidence interval plots in the case report.

Data

Use this data set; it can also be found on the companion website, ache.org /books/6Sigma.

1.77	1.67	1.66	1.81	1.90
1.65	1.63	1.89	1.99	2.56
2.06	1.50	1.92	1.21	1.89
1.75	1.29	2.10	1.70	1.76
1.69	2.19	1.64	2.20	1.97
1.69	1.93	1.55	2.02	2.11

Analysis

Observe the scatter diagram. Remark on any special characteristics.

Observe the plots of the confidence intervals. If, when comparing the corresponding confidence intervals for the two data sets, you see substantial overlap, you have reason to believe the null hypothesis, which means that no change has taken place. On the other hand, if little or no overlap is seen, there is strong reason to believe that a change has occurred. If the confidence intervals overlap substantially, not enough information is in hand to make a crisp decision.

The confidence intervals will be smaller if a lower confidence level is used. (Try it and see!) Because the confidence intervals are smaller, the confidence intervals for two samples are less likely to overlap. What does that mean about the two samples?

Lessons Learned

You are now proficient in preparing and analyzing process tracking charts; you have calculated confidence intervals for sample set averages and standard deviations.

CASE 3: PERFORMANCE EVALUATION

Topic: Six Sigma Limit Checks and Performance Ratios

In case 1, system limits were calculated on the basis of the data set for that case. In case 2, new data were gathered that appeared to show some drift and some change from case 1. Now we will analyze this change and attempt to establish whether the change is significant.

If the underlying process has drifted away from its prior condition, the process may be in jeopardy of violating the system limits, so in this exercise we will check to see if the old system limits from case 1 are still being respected. If not, new system limits will have to be issued, which will perturb the rest of the organization.

While we are at it, we will introduce two new statistical terms just so you will have seen them at least once.

Work

1. The companion website, ache.org/books/6Sigma, has the data from cases 1 and 2 organized into one long column for case 3. If you cannot access the

website at this time, copy the data from cases 1 and 2 into one long column in a new spreadsheet.

Copy the limit columns from case 1, and extend the column entries so that the plot of the limit lines will look right. Create a scatter diagram of the combined data sets and the old limits.

2. We will now see if the average value has drifted more than 1.5 standard deviations away from its original value. Six Sigma allows for this much drift in the average value. This can be done in two ways. First, calculate the change in the average value between the case 1 data and the case 2 data. Compare this change with 1.5 times the standard deviation from case 1.

The present upper system limit is drawn six standard deviations above the average using the data from case 1. Compare the average from case 2 with the upper system limit minus 4.5 times the standard deviation from case 1. Does this give the same result as the comparison just above? (Hint: It should!)

Include your conclusions in the case report. If you can figure out a graphical way to present the information, so much the better.

3. Traditional statistical process control has performance ratios that you should calculate once, just to become familiar with these terms. They are not needed elsewhere in this book, but they do appear in the literature from time to time.

The first is called the performance ratio, the symbol for which is C_p. This is defined as the system limit band divided by six times the sample standard deviation. For a well-behaved Six Sigma process, this ratio should be approximately 2.0. Calculate this for the sample set for case 1 and again for the sample set for case 2. Include the results in the case report.

4. The second traditional performance ratio is a proximity limit called $C_{p,k}$. Calculate the spacing between the sample average value and the closer system limit, then divide this by three times the sample standard deviation. For a well-behaving Six Sigma process, the ratio should be greater than 1.5.

Do this for the sample set for case 1 and again for the sample data set for case 2. Include the results in the case report.

Data

This case uses the data sets from cases 1 and 2. These data are tabulated for case 3 in the workbook found on the companion website at ache.org/books/6Sigma.

Analysis

If a substantial number of data sets were in hand, a new tracking chart could be made that would track the average sample set value. Such charts are often called

X-bar charts, with X-bar meaning the average value for each sample set. What utility would such a tracking chart, which tracks average values, provide? What limit lines should a tracking chart for the average value use? Why? (Hint: What allowance is made in Six Sigma for drift in the average value?)

Suppose the tracking chart were not merely of the sample set average values but also of confidence intervals on the sample set average values, shown perhaps as bars on the tracking chart. What utility would such a tracking chart provide? What limits should this chart use? Why?

Include your remarks in the case report. (Hint: Six Sigma does not make any allowance for drift in the standard deviation.)

Lessons Learned

You have now mastered scatter diagram manipulation and data tracking. You also have applied the Six Sigma proximity limit analysis and the classic process performance ratio analysis.

CASE 4: POTENTIAL PROBLEM ANALYSIS

Topic: No-Stick Syringe Trial

This case applies potential problem analysis. For this exercise, we will consider a new technology—namely, a certain type of no-stick syringe. The organization has become concerned about blood contamination and contagion possibilities caused by traditional syringes that rely on the administrator's control to prevent inadvertent skin punctures. Vendors have proposed new syringe designs with features that make needle sticks unlikely—but not impossible. These seem to be more cumbersome and perhaps more awkward to use because they have a surrounding structure encompassing the actual syringe, and they cost more, too. Still, needle sticks are a concern, and investigation of better devices is worthwhile.

Your organization has selected one product for trial. Your organization has not conducted any previous trial of new syringes, so there is no immediate basis for guessing what problems will arise in the trial. As project analyst, you will gather input and present a potential problem analysis. Your purpose is twofold. First, you must identify the potential problems. Second, you need to consider modifications to the trial plan to mitigate some of the potential problems.

Work

1. Create a potential problem analysis diagram. Identify at least four kinds of potential problems. Make a bulleted list of concerns for each kind of potential problem.
2. Improve the analysis by gathering input from others. If that is not workable, put yourself in the role of purchasing agent and think about the issues from the purchasing agent's perspective. Repeat in the role of the patient care unit nurse, the emergency nurse, the surgeon, and so on.
3. Propose at least one change to the trial to mitigate one or more of the potential problems.
4. Include the potential problem analysis diagram in the case report.
5. Include at least one bulleted list of details for each of the types of problems.
6. Include the recommended trial change in the case report.

Data

No data are required for this case.

Analysis

What level of detail should the potential problem analysis include? What parties are included in the development of the potential problem analysis? What should the analyst do if a potential problem comes to light that is so great as to cast the project in doubt?

Lessons Learned

You have considered the potential problems arising from a typical technology change in a healthcare organization, gathered input from others, and recommended an improvement in the trial of the new technology to mitigate a potential problem.

CASE 5: YIELD

Topic: Cumulative Process Performance

In this exercise, you will calculate results over several stages of service. The goal of the organization is to make sure everything is done right the first time. Expressed quantitatively, this is called the *first-time-through yield*.

When errors are few, counting errors is easier than counting successes. The error rate is the error count divided by the total number of opportunities for error. Yield is then defined as the complement of the error rate (the error rate subtracted from one); an error rate of 0.1 percent means a yield of 99.9 percent.

This can be seen by counting lost units. Suppose we start with 10,000 units and two process steps, each of which has an error rate of 0.1 percent and, therefore, a yield of 99.9 percent. The first process step loses 0.1 percent of 10,000 units, which is equal to 10 units. The second step loses 0.1 percent of 9,990 units, which is 9.99 units. The total loss is 19.99 units; we will call it 20. So, the overall yield is 10,000 minus the losses—in this case, 9,980. As a fraction of the starting quantity, the yield is 99.8 percent.

For low error rates, the error rates for several stages can be added together without appreciable loss of precision in the result. For example, in the two-step case above, the difference between a precise calculation and simply adding up the per-stage error rate is the difference between 19.99 and 20.00; this is negligible.

If there are five stages and the overall error rate goal is 3.4 per million, the error rate per stage must average only one-fifth of 3.4 per million, or about 0.7 per million. If there are ten stages of service, the per-stage error rate must be all the smaller, at 0.34 per million.

When selecting projects for improvement, the eye is drawn to those stages of service that contribute most of the total error. For any such improvement, the goal should be to get the error rate for that stage down to its proper share of the organization's error rate allowance or better.

Work

1. An organization finds that its accounting system enters into the service process many times. The accounting system error rate is 25 errors per million transactions, and there are 200 accounting transactions in the typical patient's record. What is the number of accounting errors to be expected in one patient's account? (Hint: Multiply the error rate by the number of opportunities for error. Remember to divide by one million,

because the error rate is given per million. The result is the expected number of errors per patient.)

2. Considering the rest of the treatment as one lumped-together stage with an error rate of seven per million opportunities, and estimating that there are an average of 500 opportunities for error in the average patient's treatment, what is the number of treatment errors to be expected in one patient's treatment?

3. What is the composite error rate, considering both accounting and treatment? (Hint: Add together the two error results from above, noting that both are stated as expected errors per patient. This sum will be the composite expected errors per patient.)

4. What is the likelihood that any one patient will have neither an accounting error nor a treatment error? (Hint: Try one minus the likelihood of having one error or the other.) This is the first-time-through yield. We ignore the effect of any one patient's account having more than one error because the error rate is small.

5. Standard deviations are determined like the sides of a triangle: by adding their squares and taking the square root of the sum. Suppose the standard deviation of the two kinds of error is two errors per million accounting transactions and three errors per million treatment opportunities. What is the standard deviation of the composite for any patient? (Hint: Multiply these per-unit values by the number of transactions of each type to get the values per patient, then add the squares and take the square root of the result.)

6. Using these results, and considering a sample of 1,000 patients, what is the number of patients expected to have no accounting errors and no treatment errors? (Hint: Multiply the first-time-through yield by the population being considered.) What is the standard deviation of this number? (Hint: Do the same with the standard deviation.)

7. State the Six Sigma system limits that apply to the overall service process. (Hint: Remember that the system limits are six standard deviations away from the average and that, in this case, the average is the first-time-through yield. If the upper system limit exceeds 100 percent, set it at 100 percent, as a yield above 100 percent is physically impossible.)

Data

No additional data are required for this case. The companion website, ache.org /books/6Sigma, has a worksheet that may be helpful when carrying out the analysis.

Analysis

The goal is to drive the error rate down below 3.4 per million; however, it may not be within the capability of the present system to meet the goal. The system limits are a conservative statement of what the present system can do. If the system is improved, the system limits can be tightened, but it is not rational to expect the present system to do better than what the system limits portray.

Does the first-time-through yield fall within the system limits? If the accounting transaction rate were reduced by a factor of ten, would that make an appreciable difference in the overall system performance? Estimate one or two pairs of error rates that would give an overall yield of 99.9997 percent because that would demonstrate Six Sigma performance.

Lessons Learned

You have now computed the yield for a two-stage service process and can readily extend this to any number of stages. You will have reflected on the difference between the goal of 3.4 errors per million and the capability of the present system as characterized by the system limits.

CASE 6: TEST RELIABILITY

Topic: Interpreting Measured Values

In this exercise, we will apply two-stage yield analysis to testing. Instruments can give the right output, but they can also give a false-positive or a false-negative output. This is of greatest concern when an instrument is set to monitor a condition and to activate an alarm or warning when a measured parameter violates a range limit. Both false conditions are worrisome because a false-negative condition means the alarm function is defeated, and a false-positive condition means confidence in the alarm system will wane.

If the instrument is directly monitoring an important process, such as the patient's temperature, the error rate is simply that of the instrument itself. If the instrument is monitoring a machine that is performing a function, and if both the machine and the instrument are subject to error, analysis needs to take into consideration the error rates of both the machine and the instrument.

Suppose the machine is a tester that looks at blood samples and declares whether or not the blood is type O+ and then produces two streams, one of declared O+ and the other of declared *not* O+. The machine can make two types of error: one is the false-positive error of declaring a sample to be O+ when in fact it is not; the other is the false-negative error of declaring a sample to be not O+ when in fact it is.

Because the point of the machine is to produce a stream of samples that the machine thinks are O+, we will pay attention to that stream and ignore the other stream of samples that the machine thinks are not O+. We will call the former the machine-selected stream, and we will not talk about the other stream at all.

The machine-selected stream will contain some number of samples that should not be there because in fact the machine made an error in letting them in. We will call this the machine's error rate, which is also the false-positive error rate.

Because this is an important matter, we will test this machine-selected stream with a tester. The tester does the same sort of examination again, testing whether the samples in this stream are indeed O+ in the tester's opinion. What we want this tester to be particularly good at is picking out samples that are not in fact O+ and rejecting them. If it rejects some good O+ samples, too, that is unfortunate, but it is tolerable.

We will divide the machine-selected stream into two fictional streams, one of true O+ samples and one of false O+ samples, so we can consider how the tester treats each kind of sample. The tester will have a distinct error rate for each kind of sample, so it is convenient to pretend there are two samples, each entirely composed of good O+ or bad O+ samples. With this leap of imagination, we can draw a diagram.

Of greatest concern is the possibility that the not-O+ sample will go through the tester, the tester will make a false-positive finding, and the sample will be accepted as if it were an O+ sample. The final output stream will consist of these hopefully few not-O+ samples plus the true O+ samples. The tester will also falsely reject some number of true O+ samples by making a false-negative finding.

Let us use some error rate parameters for the tester and see what the outcomes are:

	Blood Sample Tester	
Stream Contains	False-Positive Rate	False-Negative Rate
True O+ samples		5 per 1,000
False O+ samples	3 per 1,000	

Suppose the original machine had a false-positive rate of eight per thousand. Now we have a two-stage process, and we have all the parameters necessary to calculate the makeup of the output stream that is supposed to contain almost entirely true O+ samples. Of those samples identified as O+ after the test and the check, how many are really O+? Because the error rate of the checking instrument appears to be worse than the error rate of the machine, one may suspect that the checking may do more harm than good.

The work in the next section involves a lot of opportunities for getting the wrong factor in the wrong place. The safe way to proceed is to draw a diagram as in exhibit 11.1.

As in exhibit 11.1, show the tester on the left with two output streams: one correct and one false. Connect the "correct" line to a checker box, which itself has two outputs: true positive and false negative. Connect the "false" line to a separate checker box, which itself has two outputs: true negative and false positive. Write the fractions next to each line. Write the calculated values on the diagram as they are produced so that you can keep track of the results.

Exhibit 11.1: O+ Machine and Tester

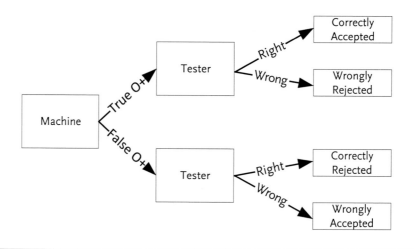

Work

1. Using the machine false-positive error rate and the tester false-positive rate, calculate the composite error rate. (Hint: Refer to case 5.) This is the impurity rate in the final O+ stream.
2. Calculate the machine's yield, which is 100 percent minus the false-positive error rate. Use this value and the tester's false-negative rate to calculate the fraction of the stream that is falsely rejected by the tester.

3. Refer to exhibit 11.1, which shows the tester with two input streams and four output streams. In the previous two steps, you have calculated the stream fractions for two of the four output streams. Now calculate the other two so that all of the input flow will be accounted for in the output flows.
4. Include a diagram in your report. On the diagram, enter the output stream fractions.

Data

The error rates for the machine and the tester are given above.

Analysis

What is the purity of the final stream of O+ samples? How does this compare with the purity rate of the samples coming out of the machine? Does the tester improve the purity of the output stream? If so, what is the reduction in the impurity achieved by the tester stage?

Suppose it is physically possible to add a second tester downstream of the present tester, and suppose the error rates of the second tester are the same as those of the present tester. How much further improvement, if any, would you expect to be achieved by an added stage of testing?

At each stage of testing, some of the product is lost to false negatives. How would you trade off the additional purity achieved by additional testing against product loss due to false negatives?

Lessons Learned

You have observed by now that, although the arithmetic in this kind of analysis is not very complicated, the opportunity for confusion is great. Drawing a diagram is good practice.

You have just analyzed a complex two-stage process and computed the effective yield of this process. You will have seen that the practice of drawing out processes in simple diagrams is rewarding because it clarifies thinking and captures that thinking in a useful way. More complex systems can be analyzed in this way, provided a suitable diagram can be drawn.

CASE 7: TIME-VALUE CHARTS

Topic: Comparing Two Scenarios

Time-value charts are helpful tools for analyzing multistep problems, especially those involving delays of various kinds. Draw a line, starting at the left side of the page, and move the pencil to the right to represent a period of time. If no value is being added during that time, the line runs horizontally. If some value is being added, the line rises on a slope so that the rise is proportional to the value added. Precision in time is usually more important than precision in value.

For this example, consider that a certain medical book is to be ordered online or purchased at the nearest university bookstore. Suppose the price will be about the same either way.

Work

1. Draw a time-value line for the online purchase scenario.
2. Draw a second time-value line for the trip to the university bookstore.
3. Include both lines in the project report.
4. Repeat steps 1 and 2, this time considering the matter from the point of view of your organization, and consider the fact that time spent by you away from your station is a negative value to your organization. Buying the book, however, is a positive value to your organization.

Data

No additional data are required for this case.

Analysis

Consider which of the strategies is better from each of the two points of view; include any other observations.

This technique is also useful for analyzing multistep processes from the point of view of the patient and of the healthcare organization. Indeed, there may be several different points of view in practical situations. The sketch can bring these viewpoints to light and, perhaps, help reconcile conflicting interests.

Lessons Learned

You have analyzed time-value sketches from two points of view and used these as simple devices to explain a multistep process.

CASE 8: THE POISSON DISTRIBUTION

Topic: Discrete Events Modeling

The normal distribution gets the most use, but other distributions are of practical interest as well. This case considers the Poisson distribution, which applies to discrete events, each of low probability. Experience shows that the Poisson distribution applies to the number of telephone calls attempted during a busy hour, the number of patrons showing up at a bank branch at lunchtime, the number of people arriving to use an automatic teller machine at mid-afternoon on Friday, and so on.

These scenarios are important because service organizations cannot possibly design themselves to serve their clients if every one of the clients shows up at once. A bank may have 10,000 depositors, and if all of them show up at once, the bank is going to be swamped. In addition, the bank cannot possibly construct a building big enough to take care of a surge of 10,000 customers. Because 100 percent capacity is not going to be provided, what should be the basis for some reasonable level of capacity?

The immediate follow-up question is, what is to be done if a surge in demand exceeds the service capacity provided? If these surges are sufficiently rare, the organization can plead that all reasonable measures were already taken. If the surges are not sufficiently rare, the client population may look elsewhere for service.

The Poisson distribution also applies to trial evaluations when errors are of low probability. If the expected number of errors per 1,000 events is three, what should be considered if the observed error rate is zero? Or four?

The Poisson distribution has one odd feature: The standard deviation and the average are not independent of each other the way they are in the normal distribution. Instead, the standard deviation is the square root of the average value for the Poisson distribution.

The Poisson distribution does not have the bell-curve profile seen in common applications; rather, it has a steeper slope on the left-hand side and a less steep slope on the right-hand side. The curve stops at the origin because a negative number of discrete events has no meaning. The Poisson distribution does take on the familiar bell shape if the average is a large number, but that is not the range of interest or purpose when the Poisson distribution is being applied.

Sometimes it is of interest to check the distribution to find out how likely it is that a particular number of events will occur. More often, there is a range of numbers of interest given the question, "What range of occurrences might one expect with 95 percent confidence?" With that answer, the organization can establish a capacity to deal with 95 percent of the occurrences and have a defendable position. The 95 percent value is a confidence level; if the organization has the matching capacity, the organization, with 95 percent confidence, can handle the traffic. The 95 percent value is also called a "service level" when it is used to size capacity.

For this case, consider an emergency department located near a metalworking factory that employs 2,000 workers and where workers get burned badly enough to require care 12 times a month, on average. The number varies from month to month and seems to follow a Poisson distribution, as indeed it should if the burns result from random accidents in the course of work. The maximum number of cases might be 2,000 if every worker got burned. To provide capacity to treat 2,000 cases would seem to be rash, given that the average number is only 12. What is a reasonable number of cases to use as the planning basis?

Work

1. Open a spreadsheet and create a column of numbers running from 0 to 25. In the adjacent column, enter the Poisson distribution values, or ordinates, for the average value of 12. In the next column, do the same, but enter the cumulative Poisson distribution for each of the numbers in the first column. In Excel, the Poisson function is POISSON(x, mean, cumulative?). (Note that Excel 2016 actually has two identical functions—POISSON[. . .] and POISSON.DIST[. . .]—but the former is used throughout the book for simplicity.) The x value is the number in the first column; the mean is the average value, namely 12; and the third argument is "false" for the ordinate column and "true" for the cumulative column. The cumulative column sums up all the values from zero to the present number. (Hint: Be sure to start counting from zero, not from one.)
2. Create a chart of the ordinate column, which will look a little like a bell curve but will not be symmetric.
3. Create a chart of the third column, which will be an S-curve rising to near unity.

4. Include both charts in the report.
5. What is the likelihood of having exactly ten burns in a month? (Hint: Read the ordinate column.)
6. What fraction of the total possibilities will be ten or fewer cases in a month? (Hint: Read the cumulative column.)
7. What number is so large that 95 percent of all possibilities will be that number or less? (Hint: Work backward from the cumulative column.) What about for 90 percent?

Data

The primary datum needed for this exercise is that the average value is 12.

Analysis

Experiment with different average values; try 4, and try 25. You will see that the distribution is quite skewed for the average value of 4 and much like a bell curve for 25. For large average values, not much distinction is seen between the normal curve and the Poisson curve, so it is not rash to take advantage of the convenience of using the normal curve in many cases, even where the Poisson curve might be better justified from a theoretical basis.

Excel does not provide an inverse Poisson function, so it is necessary to generate the list of cumulative values to get the argument corresponding to, say, 95 percent.

In your report, recommend a service level, and recommend the matching capacity requirement for burn treatments starting with the average case rate of 12 per month. Defend your recommendations.

Lessons Learned

You just analyzed a discrete event of low probability using the Poisson distribution, which is useful in sizing capacities to serve large populations, not all of whom are expected to need the service at the same time. You also have applied a service level to establish the capacity plan.

CASE 9: INCOMPLETE TRIALS

Topic: Cumulative Analysis

In this exercise, we will deal with incomplete trials by analyzing cumulative data. A trial often produces incomplete information. For instance, if 20 people join a trial but 4 of them are reassigned during the trial period and therefore do not complete their part, 20 percent of the potential data will not be available. Although this can be dealt with by accepting a reduced data set or starting with extra participants to allow for some shrinkage, it is helpful to have some technique for dealing with the incomplete data in a systematic way. There is such a technique for duration testing, which is also called life testing.

1. Start with a population of samples to be tested for lifetime. For those that reach the end state, collect the data. For those that do not reach the end state, note the time at which they dropped out of the test.
2. Sort the data so the longest-lived is first and the shortest-lived is last, including the dropouts. Highlight the dropouts to distinguish them from the others.
3. Count the data points. Note the top 10 percent, the top 20 percent, and so on through the top 90 percent. For example, if there were 50 items at the start and 10 dropped out, the top 10 percent is the top 5 items.
4. A reasonable confidence interval on the lifetime can then be read directly from these results, with the 90 percent confidence interval corresponding to the top 90 percent result. This is necessarily conservative because the dropouts could not have had a shorter lifetime than their dropout time.

If the population is large, the confidence intervals can be improved somewhat by fitting the data to the cumulative distribution of the most likely model, such as a bathtub curve. If the population has 20 or fewer members, the uncertainty in the fit outweighs any gain from the modeling.

Consider this scenario. A trial gets under way to test the value, utility, and user satisfaction of pocket-sized computers for use by orderlies in a long-term care facility. As the analyst, you note that a potential problem is battery lifetime. No information is available that would help you gauge lifetime; however, if the trial is successful and computers are subsequently issued to all employees, you'll need some estimate of lifetime so that you can plan for replacement units. Therefore, you arrange to collect data on battery lifetime as an adjunct to the trial.

During the trial, various things happen. Some computers get damaged and are removed from the trial. Two of the people using the computers in the trial are transferred to other assignments, and they turn in their computers. At the end of the trial, you need to extract such information so that you can pull together the data gathered on battery life.

Work

1. Enter the data from the next section into a spreadsheet. (These data are already available in computer format on the companion website, ache.org/books/6Sigma.) Sort the data in descending order: Select the DATA menu, click SORT, select DESCENDING, and pick the data set for sorting.
2. Move those data that are marked "incomplete" to a second column so that, when the data are plotted, these appear in a different color. Drag and drop, using the mouse. Plot the data using horizontal bars.
3. Count off the top 10 percent, 20 percent, 50 percent, 75 percent, and 90 percent.
4. Report the 75 percent confidence lifetime (the cutoff for the top 75 percent of lifetimes). On the basis of this trial, 75 percent or more of computers put into use can expect to have a battery lifetime at least this long.

Data

ID	Life	Event	ID	Life	Event
A	24.0	OK	K	27.0	OK
B	10.0	OK	L	21.5	OK
C	16.5	OK	M	11.0	OK
D	20.0	Broken	N	28.0	OK
E	25.5	OK	O	19.5	Broken
F	28.5	OK	P	19.0	OK
G	18.5	OK	Q	17.6	OK
H	16.0	OK	R	19.0	OK
I	13.0	Quit	S	18.0	OK
J	17.5	Quit	T	19.0	OK

The lifetime is quoted in days. The event is marked "OK" if the event was a normal battery replacement. These data can also be found on the companion website, ache.org/books/6Sigma.

Analysis

Consider what would happen to this analysis if half the participants dropped out after five days. (Hint: What would happen to the 75 percent cutoff?) Consider what would happen if the not-OK items were simply deleted from the study. Would the 75 percent cutoff go up or down? Note that no assumption is made in this analysis about the nature of the distribution function governing battery lifetime. The procedure simply ranks the outcomes without trying to find any parameters for functions.

Like all statistical methods of analysis, this procedure is weak if the data sample set is small. Even so, if only a few data samples are available, this procedure is better than nothing, and it makes productive use of even the defective data samples.

Lessons Learned

You have now analyzed lifetime data samples, including defective samples, to estimate confidence intervals for studies of lifetimes.

CASE 10: FAILURE MODES AND EFFECTS

Topic: Linkages

Failures happen. The systematic analysis of failures is necessary to prevent recurrence. This book has dealt with chains of events, fishbone diagrams, and failure modes and effects analysis. All of these are useful, and all seek to portray the linkages among actions, events, and consequences. Of these, failure modes and effects analysis deals directly with failure analysis. Something failed. Something might fail. What happens then?

A failure modes and effects analysis can be done to any depth. For example, say that a part broke. What factors might have caused the part to break? And what might have caused the *factors* themselves? These linkages can be drawn out in an ever-expanding tree. Proceeding in the other direction, if the part fails, what result occurs? And what happens as a consequence of that result? Again, you can build another ever-expanding tree. Generally, it is useful to carry out failure modes and effects analysis for at least two steps in each direction. The nature of the particular event will then dictate whether further expansion would be helpful.

In drawing out the tree, it is customary to reserve judgment about which branch is the most likely until the tree is drawn out sufficiently. At that point, judgment and experience can usually narrow down the branches of interest, with the others held in reserve.

In this case, suppose that a healthcare organization provides bed care for patients and that, in recent months, three patients have fallen out of bed during nighttime hours. Each bed has rails, each patient has access to a call button with an attendant on call, and there is a step stool beside each bed. In short, the system was designed to prevent the very falls now being observed.

Because more than one patient is involved, there must be a system problem. Linking relationships between the effect (a fallen patient) and the possible causes (the failure[s] of the prevention devices) may be illuminating.

Work

1. Draw a failure modes and effects tree to portray the linkage between the prevention devices and the event. Carry the tree out to three or four stages. Use separate sheets as necessary for legibility. Include the tree or trees in the report.
2. Identify the two or three most likely problems, using your own judgment. Form a hypothesis as to the most likely cause. Include the hypothesis in the report.
3. Identify additional data that would be required to validate the hypothesis. Include the data list in the report, perhaps in summary form.
4. Identify a test or trial program that would provide the validation data. Include recommendations in the report.

Data

No additional data are required for this case.

Analysis

The most common benefit of such analysis is to organize the thinking of a work group to forestall any jumping to conclusions. For this reason alone, a failure modes and effects analysis is often worthwhile.

In situations like this case, one often finds that the system had preventive measures in place that would have worked—had they not been defeated by the patient, a visitor, or staff. Designing preventive measures that cannot be defeated is an ongoing challenge. Alarms and monitoring systems, such as one that could detect whether a bed rail is up, are an interesting design problem, and perhaps a good solution will arise that will provide a practicable solution.

Lessons Learned

You have now applied failure modes and effects analysis to a practical problem.

CASE 11: DISCRETE ANALYSIS

Topic: Known Populations

In some cases, the total population of interest is known and can be counted. If so, specific methods apply. Consider the following case. The organization has a number of gurneys for moving patients around the building. The gurneys are to be returned to the gurney pool at the end of each use, and some data gathering shows that any one gurney is at the pool location 40 percent of the time. The organization has considered how many gurneys need to be on hand in the pool at any time and has established a policy that, with 90 percent confidence, at least seven gurneys must always be at the pool location to take care of surges in demand.

The department manager identifies two possible approaches. One is to hire a gurney wrangler to walk the floors and bring back orphaned gurneys the way grocery stores hire shopping cart wranglers to round up carts in parking lots. The second option is to buy more gurneys, if the right number to buy can be determined.

For a fixed population of gurneys, the likelihood that at least seven will be in the pool can be calculated using the binomial distribution. The binomial distribution applies when exactly two states are possible: In this case, the gurney is either in the pool or it is not. Thus, the binomial distribution applies. (If there were three or more possibilities, another distribution, the multinomial, would apply.)

The binomial distribution requires the following input: the target count, the total population count, and the probability. If the total population of gurneys were 12 and the probability 40 percent, the confidence level for finding *at least* 7 gurneys in the pool would be the sum of the likelihoods of finding 7, 8, 9, 10, 11, or 12 gurneys in the pool.

The likelihood of *not* finding at least seven gurneys in the pool would be the sum of the likelihoods of finding zero, one, two, three, four, five, or six in the pool. The sum of the two likelihoods (finding and not finding at least seven gurneys in the pool) must be 100 percent. The binomial distribution looks like the normal distribution for most sets of parameters. It is available as a built-in function in Excel and in other spreadsheet applications.

Work

1. Open a spreadsheet. Create a column of numbers running from 0 to 12. (Hint: Be sure to include 0.) Label this the "Count" column; this corresponds to the number of gurneys in the pool at any one time.
2. In the next column, compute the corresponding binomial distribution values given a total population of 12 and a probability of 40 percent. Use BINOM.DIST(count, population size, probability, false). The "false" entry tells the function to return the distribution value or ordinate rather than the cumulative distribution.
3. Plot the distribution.
4. In a third column, compute for each count in the first column the cumulative binomial distribution by using BINOM.DIST(count, population size, true). Plot these values.
5. Returning to the question of how many gurneys should be in the population to have at least 7 in the pool given that the probability of any 1 gurney being in the pool is 40 percent, note that BINOM.DIST(6, 17, 40%, true) would return the likelihood of 6 or fewer gurneys being in the pool if the total population is 17. Because what is wanted is not that but rather the opposite, the desired result will be returned by calculating 1 minus BINOM.DIST(6, 17, 40%, true).
6. Create a column of population sizes running from 12 to 40. Fill in the next column using the values found for 1 minus BINOM.DIST(6, population size, probability, true). This column is, for each population size, the likelihood of having seven or more gurneys in the pool. Plot these points.
7. From the previous steps, select the population size that would give 90 percent confidence that at least 7 gurneys will be in the pool. Include this in the report.

Data

No additional data are required for this case.

Analysis

How much would the confidence level improve if five additional gurneys were acquired? How much would the confidence level fall if five fewer gurneys were taken away from the pool?

In analyzing the potential problems that might arise if this policy is followed, the analyst considers that people might be less diligent in returning gurneys to the pool if there are more of them on hand. Suppose the in-pool probability drops to 35 percent. How much would the confidence level drop then? How many more gurneys would be needed to make up for the drop in in-pool probability? Consider these matters for inclusion in the report.

Lessons Learned

You have just performed a service improvement analysis using discrete analysis. In doing this, you have considered the importance of incremental changes in the population size and in the probability parameter.

CASE 12: CENTRAL LIMIT THEOREM

Topic: Central Tendency

Nature sides with the bell-shaped curve. The normal distribution is used in statistical analysis both for convenience and to take advantage of a powerful central tendency captured in the central limit theorem. This theorem states that estimates of the average value will be distributed by the normal distribution with the same average value as that of the underlying population and that the standard deviation of the sample average will be equal to the standard deviation of the underlying population divided by the square root of the sample size as the total number of samples grows to a large number.

So, if the underlying population is, say, Poisson, the distribution of sample averages from this distribution will be the normal distribution. If the underlying population is binomial, the distribution of sample averages from this distribution will be the normal distribution. The same is true for any underlying population. (The theorem requires the standard deviation of the underlying population be finite, which is always true in real situations.)

The standard deviation of the sample average will drop to zero as the sample size grows, so the sample average will be known more and more precisely as the sample size grows. This theorem applies even if the sample average being tracked is the sum of samples drawn from various distributions.

The practical effect of this remarkable theorem is that any sample average can be modeled using the normal distribution. Because almost any parameter being observed is the result of several subprocesses acting to give an accumulated result, that observed parameter is going to behave according to the normal distribution. Thus, it is a reasonable practice in the real world to presume that the normal distribution applies unless a clear indication exists to think otherwise.

This case will demonstrate the central limit theorem by drawing samples from the uniform distribution, which is handily available in Excel as a built-in function. The uniform distribution returns a result between 0 and 1, with all numbers in between being equally likely. This is not a bell curve; it is a flat line. The Excel function is RAND(). Other spreadsheet applications use similar but different names. RAND() is a volatile function, so every time the sheet is recalculated, the value returned by RAND() changes. Test this by hitting the F9 key, which forces a recalculation of the page. Repeat this several times.

To freeze the value, do the following. Select the cells to be frozen. From the EDIT menu, select COPY. The menu will now disappear. Select EDIT again, then choose PASTE SPECIAL, and then select VALUES on the panel. Close the menu. This writes the values into the same cells in which RAND() had been located. This process is destructive, so if you want to generate the RAND() results again, it is necessary to retype the RAND() formulae. An in-between approach is to copy the frozen values onto a different sheet so that the formulae are preserved.

Work

1. Open a spreadsheet. Make a column of 20 entries, all of them being equal to RAND(). Note that the cells all have different values, even though the cell formulae are all the same. Hit F9 a few times to cause the sheet to be recalculated. Note that the values in the column are volatile.
2. Freeze the values. Copy the values onto a new spreadsheet or onto a blank part of the same spreadsheet, using the PASTE SPECIAL/VALUES procedure explained earlier. Create a histogram of these frozen values using a small bin size. (Refer back to cases 1, 2, and 3 to refresh your memory regarding bins and histograms.) Plot the histogram. Remark in the report whether this distribution appears to be more or less uniform.

3. Return to the sheet with the column of random numbers. Copy the column several times so that the sheet will have 50 columns of 20 rows, all being samples from the uniform distribution. Calculate the average and standard deviation for the whole set of 1,000 cells. Report your results.

4. For each of the 20 columns, compute the average. Make a histogram of these set averages. Plot the results. Note for the report whether the distribution of these set averages appears to be uniform, bell-shaped, or other. (Hint: The central limit theorem suggests the distribution will be the normal distribution.)

5. Force recalculation of the sheet by hitting F9 a few times. Note whether the plot of averages changes with each recalculation. Note whether the histogram of averages changes. (Hint: The histogram does not update itself automatically. To force an update, use the TOOLS menu/DATA ANALYSIS/ HISTOGRAM procedure.) Report your findings.

Data

No additional data are required for this case.

Analysis

Before computers were on every desk, random numbers were published in large books. Books of normally distributed random numbers were generated by adding up seven random numbers drawn from the uniform distribution, which was a direct application of the central limit theorem. All cumulative distributions are uniform between zero and unity, by definition. Therefore, it is possible to create a random number generator for any distribution for which an inverse function is at hand. For example, Excel provides an inverse function for the normal distribution, so a normally distributed random-number generator can be written by the formula =NORM. INV(RAND[], AVERAGE, STANDARD DEVIATION) for any specified average value and standard deviation. Try a column of these with the average value of zero and standard deviation of one. The cells will all have the formula =NORM.INV(RAND[],0,1). Hit F9 a few times to force a recalculation so that you can see the dynamic. Create and plot a histogram. Does this look like a normal distribution?

Lessons Learned

By manipulating random numbers from the uniform distribution, you have demonstrated the validity of the central limit theorem. You generated normally distributed random numbers in two ways: by directly applying the central limit theorem and by combining built-in spreadsheet functions.

CASE 13: DATA SAMPLING

Topic: Reduced Tracking Methods

One way to reduce effort is by sampling the data. Analysis of a partial data set—that is, a sample—works fine if the sample is a high-fidelity representation of the underlying population. If a lot of data are available to start with, as might be the case when analyzing past data that happens to be at hand, random sampling can be used. Suppose there are 100 patient records, and you want to look at 10 of them. Open a spreadsheet, make a column that goes from 1 to 100, make a second column of random numbers, freeze the random numbers, and then sort the table in order of descending random numbers. Take the case numbers from the top ten rows of the sorted table. You now have ten randomly selected cases.

For ongoing projects, it is usually difficult to organize activities so that data are taken at random. Taking temperatures at the end of a shift is not done at random; taking temperatures after meals is not done at random. Either of these processes may be fine for other purposes, but they are not random samples of a patient's temperature over the entirety of the day. Alternatively, it is not likely to be rewarding to wake a patient up at three o'clock in the morning to get a temperature sample just to conform to a random-interval sampling plan.

Practicable data sampling for ongoing projects is likely to be periodic: once a shift, once a day, or once every hour. For this example, we will look at the once-an-hour sampling plan. If the underlying process has a component that also varies slowly, this may be a good periodic sampling plan. On the other hand, if the underlying process varies rapidly or has brief episodes, this plan will miss important features of the data. A good understanding of the process being sampled is necessary.

How should you proceed? Past experience is an excellent guide. However, if no past experience is available, start sampling frequently, observe the data, and extend the sampling period gradually.

The act of sampling presents opportunities for error in reading and transcribing the sample values. To the extent that these are random, they do not matter much unless the data set is very small. If they are not random because, say, a gauge is read from an angle to one side so that the readings always err on the low side, a bias introduces itself into the process. If estimation is required, the reading error can be quite substantial. For example, an estimate of a patient's weight is not likely to be very precise.

Work

1. Organize the data in the next section into one long column on a spreadsheet; the data can also be found on the companion website, ache.org/books/6Sigma. Compute the average value and the standard deviation. Create a histogram with some reasonable bin size to visualize the data. Select some information for the report.

2. Try a periodic sampling plan—say, every tenth row—and make a new column with this sample set. One way to have the spreadsheet do this is to create a counter column that gives the row number. Set the sample spacing in a cell. In the sample data column, write a formula such as =IF(MOD[counter, spacing]=0, neighboring value from full set, 0). Once you have the sample set, compute its parameters. Then compute the 90 percent confidence intervals on the sample average and sample standard deviation. Perform a T.TEST(. . .) and an F.TEST(. . .) to compare the sample set and the original set. Create a histogram. Form an opinion on the goodness of the fit of the sampling plan.

3. Repeat these steps with some other sampling plans. Select one or two parameters as good measures of the sampling plans and plot these. Include the plot in the report.

4. Select a sampling plan to recommend to management.

Data

This is the full data set, from which reduced samples are to be drawn; it can also be found on the companion website, ache.org/books/6Sigma.

Full Data Set				
14.34	16.46	12.23	19.17	17.41
17.60	12.39	16.71	16.78	15.57
13.30	13.48	17.12	13.88	18.07
16.24	16.86	15.51	18.10	18.30
15.09	9.14	18.73	18.83	13.41
17.59	19.49	16.29	15.23	15.18
15.23	16.94	13.61	17.80	18.50

(continued)

(continued from previous page)

Full Data Set				
18.01	14.85	14.47	17.10	18.95
13.71	14.93	20.91	17.19	16.23
12.98	20.70	16.05	17.56	19.79
17.67	13.54	15.78	17.34	12.29
13.48	15.69	19.16	13.12	17.30
17.04	19.60	15.81	15.98	19.22
19.35	17.34	14.60	19.52	12.73
10.21	16.73	19.89	13.65	16.35
15.82	18.35	14.51	15.28	19.13
17.01	14.69	14.44	18.74	15.12
17.12	13.36	19.28	11.37	14.61
16.40	17.87	18.47	14.63	18.82
19.43	15.08	13.91	20.19	15.99
17.11	14.00	15.01	14.87	18.30
14.22	14.88	16.19	17.84	15.45
18.71	17.97	16.52	16.53	11.92
15.84	15.13	18.20	16.69	14.13
15.23	15.25	16.35	15.74	16.40
19.91	16.22	17.38	19.91	13.20
16.32	14.91	18.11	15.27	17.07
18.66	17.14	13.54	14.22	18.83
16.37	14.24	16.84	17.90	15.96
17.46	19.54	15.97	17.54	12.77
18.65	20.80	15.94	18.34	20.48
16.97	14.12	14.90	18.83	14.05
17.83	12.85	17.23	13.02	17.77
15.54	15.63	15.93	16.68	17.11
18.14	14.28	16.74	18.01	14.27
15.75	15.05	18.32	15.86	14.68
17.20	14.69	16.81	20.07	21.54
14.80	17.05	15.10	16.32	14.75
16.57	15.56	20.22	15.61	11.90
14.85	17.49	11.86	15.70	18.41

Analysis

If taking more samples costs more time and effort in a linear way, so that taking twice as many samples takes twice as much effort, is there a best choice for the sampling plan? How would you address this issue? What visualizations of the original data set and any sample set give the most insight into the goodness of fit of the sample plan?

Any sampling plan would have to be run on a trial basis to confirm that it works in practice as well as it works on the blackboard. State your method for deciding how long to run such a trial. Include these findings in your report.

Lessons Learned

You have now considered random sampling to reduce data acquisition cost by testing candidate sampling plans against a full data set. You have considered classical analysis of the sample sets and visualization of the results and have considered the minimum running time for a trial to validate the selected sampling plan.

CASE 14: RULE-BASED SAMPLING

Topic: Focused Tracking Methods

It may be helpful to create a rule for when samples are to be taken. Rule-based sampling focuses attention on key times and key events, which are times when random sampling or periodic sampling would not provide sufficient insight.

When a machine is turned on, the obvious thing to do is to check it and its setup immediately to see if it is operable. Electronics are known to fail most often just when the machine is turned on, so the fact that the machine ran yesterday is not sufficient to know that it will run today. Indeed, most computerized machines check themselves upon boot-up for this very reason.

A computer self-check is limited to the computer and its slaved equipment, so a computer self-check is usually not a sufficient test of the equipment. It is necessary to verify that leads are connected properly, that any supplies are loaded in, and so on. The computer self-test is necessary, but a complete equipment checkup goes further. A functional test, which involves running the equipment against a known standard, is good practice every time any machine is turned on.

If the functional test fails, adjust the machine and try again. If the machine runs successfully for two tests, the machine is probably okay. If either of the two tests fails, the machine should be declared suspect and either replaced or repaired immediately or double-checked continually while it is being used. This is rule-based sampling. The rule in this case is to validate the machine by testing the first one or two applications after each boot-up of the machine.

Random sampling may then be used for the rest of the run, but it clearly would not be likely to catch setup errors that would affect the first several applications until the first random sample was checked. Because of this, rule-based sampling has a role to play in any system.

Rule-based sampling is commonly applied if there is a known periodic behavior or conditioned behavior and only high (or low) values are of interest. Taking temperatures after an exercise period is likely to capture the highest temperature of the day. Taking the pulse rate at three o'clock in the morning is likely to get the lowest reading of the day. Rules based on the purpose of the measurement and the known periodic or conditioned behavior provide the key information with a minimum sampling effort.

Measurements of recovery time are commonly of interest. How long does it take for respiration rate to return to normal after five minutes of exercise? The recovery follows a known law—in this case, an exponential curve—and samples taken during the recovery period can fix the parameters of the curve to sufficient precision. Other recovery processes may follow a different law (How long does it take the employee parking lot to clear out after the end of a shift?), but the law is usually pretty easy to discover by observation. If the law is known, a rule to guide any sampling can be developed in a straightforward way.

Work

1. Using data set 1 from the next section, set a rule for sampling that will give the highest readings during each cycle. Do this by picking a window of about five consecutive data points from the full data set when the readings are highest, then use the same window in the next cycle, and so on. Next, pick a sampling plan that looks into this window, by rule, and takes a sufficient number of samples from that window to have a reasonable confidence that the average of the samples is not much less than the window average in the original data set. What confidence level seems reasonable to you? How are you going to apply the confidence level in this case, when only one side of the distribution is of interest?

2. Using data set 2 that follows, which is an exponential recovery data set, pick a sampling plan that will give an average value, with reasonable confidence, for the first five minutes. From that average plus the reading at five minutes, the exponential parameter can be calculated. What confidence level seems to be reasonable?

Data

Use the following data sets; these can also be found on the companion website, ache.org/books/6Sigma.

Data set 1 includes data with a periodic component:

Data Set 1				
21.0	20.6	21.0	21.2	20.4
21.3	21.8	21.4	21.8	21.8
21.8	22.2	21.9	22.6	22.3
23.4	22.9	23.0	22.9	22.7
23.7	23.1	23.8	23.5	23.3
23.6	24.1	24.3	23.8	24.1
24.9	24.0	24.4	24.1	24.3
24.8	24.8	24.6	24.3	24.8
25.1	24.5	24.8	24.6	25.4
24.8	24.7	24.9	24.9	24.9
24.7	24.8	25.4	25.0	24.7
24.3	24.9	25.0	25.1	24.6
24.5	24.6	24.5	24.2	24.3
24.3	23.7	24.2	23.9	23.6
23.0	23.3	23.3	23.2	23.7
22.9	23.0	22.9	22.9	22.6
22.0	22.8	22.6	22.4	22.0
21.3	21.2	21.3	21.8	21.5
20.3	21.1	20.7	20.6	21.0
19.7	20.0	20.4	19.9	20.1
19.1	19.0	18.8	19.0	18.7
18.3	18.3	18.6	18.4	18.4
17.8	17.7	17.4	18.2	18.1
17.2	17.1	16.9	16.7	16.9

(continued)

(continued from previous page)

Data Set 1				
16.2	16.0	16.8	16.8	16.9
16.2	15.9	16.1	15.5	15.8
15.7	15.3	16.0	15.8	15.1
15.2	15.4	14.9	15.3	15.4
15.5	14.9	15.3	14.9	14.8
15.3	15.4	15.4	14.6	15.2
15.2	15.4	15.0	14.7	15.1
15.6	15.5	15.6	15.6	15.7

Data set 2, exponential recovery, includes the times at which the values were read:

Data Set 2: Exponential Recovery (time given in seconds)					
Time	Value	Time	Value	Time	Value
6	41.0	54	40.6	102	40.3
12	40.9	60	40.6	108	40.3
18	40.9	66	40.6	114	40.3
24	40.8	72	40.5	120	40.2
30	40.8	78	40.5	126	40.2
36	40.7	84	40.4	132	40.2
42	40.7	90	40.4	138	40.1
48	40.7	96	40.4	144	40.1
150	40.1	222	39.7	294	39.4
156	40.0	228	39.7	300	39.4
162	40.0	234	39.6	306	39.4
168	40.0	240	39.6	312	39.3
174	39.9	246	39.6	318	39.3
180	39.9	252	39.6	324	39.3
186	39.9	258	39.5	330	39.3
192	39.8	264	39.5	336	39.2
198	39.8	270	39.5	342	39.2
204	39.8	276	39.5	348	39.2
210	39.8	282	39.4	354	39.2
216	39.7	288	39.4	360	39.2

Analysis

In both of these cases, the time at which the samples are drawn may be important. Rule-based sampling plans that rely on extremely precise timing are obviously unworkable in the real world. For each of the preceding cases, estimate the effect, if any, if the readings are delayed by one time unit (one row). What if they are delayed by two time units? How many time units of delay do you estimate would be required to cause a significant error in the result?

The work instructions for these cases have not specified any visualization charts. Reports generally have some charts, so pick out one or two that would portray the essence of each analysis.

Lessons Learned

You have just developed sampling rules for periodic and exponential data sets. You have also considered the consequence of taking samples at delayed times, which has involved a departure from the original plan.

CASE 15: RICH DATA SETS

Topic: Classical Set Analysis

Much of this book has been devoted to dealing with limited data sets because, in the real world, gathering data takes time and effort. However, occasions arise that bring an ocean of data, and the task for the analyst is to deal with the flood. If the data are already in computer files, the task is simplified to applying classical statistical analysis.

For example, if delivery times for X-rays to patient care units are recorded by time stamping, and the time stamps flow into a computer file, there will be a flood of data.

Work

1. The data sets in the next section record X-ray delivery times to different locations—labeled A, B, C, and D—in the building complex. Supervisors in location D assert that their service is materially worse than what is provided to the other locations.

Start with the null hypothesis that the service to D is the same as the service to A, then repeat with D and B, and again with D and C. Follow the next steps for each pair.

2. Select a high confidence level, say 90 percent, because management is involved.

   Apply the T.TEST(. . .) for each pair (D-A, D-B, and D-C) to see if the null hypothesis is valid for the average values. The T.TEST function requires four arguments. The first two are the data sets to be compared; the remaining two establish options for the analysis. Use values 2 and 3 for these options; these values mean, respectively, that both tails are to be considered and that the data sets have unequal standard deviations. So, if the data sets are in columns E and F, rows 12 through 97, the entry would be T.TEST(E12:E97, F12:F97, 2, 3). This test returns a probability that the null hypothesis is true with regard to the average values of the data sets. Compare the result with the requirement of 90 percent confidence.

3. Apply the F.TEST(. . .) to each pair to see if the null hypothesis is valid for the standard deviation. This test returns a probability that the null hypothesis is true with regard to the standard deviations of the data sets. Compare the result with the requirement of 90 percent confidence. The F.TEST does not require any parameters, only the data sets.

4. Sort each data set one at a time. Figure out where the top 10 percent cutoff is. (Hint: Count back 10 percent of the rows from the end of the set.) This cutoff represents the time to deliver 90 percent of the deliveries to each location. Compare these times. Repeat your examination for the 75 percent and 50 percent cutoffs. Make a table of these results so that they can be compared visually.

Data

Use this data set; it can also be found on the companion website, ache.org/books/6Sigma.

Item	A	B	C	D
1	22.8	16.3	19.4	22.2
2	22.4	19.3	20.6	22.6
3	18.7	20.3	21.6	22.2
4	14.9	25.2	18.6	21.3

(continued)

(continued from previous page)

Item	A	B	C	D
5	21.7	20.7	18.5	23.1
6	18.2	15.4	20.7	21.8
7	17.7	19.3	21.8	23.0
8	20.8	19.6	20.6	21.4
9	22.7	14.9	22.6	21.8
10	19.7	20.7	22.2	22.0
11	17.0	26.4	19.6	22.9
12	19.4	17.6	23.0	21.6
13	20.0	22.7	23.6	22.2
14	19.4	24.8	17.6	21.9
15	18.8	16.4	18.6	22.0
16	21.1	19.4	16.5	22.0
17	16.6	16.5	18.1	21.2
18	18.0	16.6	19.9	21.7
19	15.8	21.9	18.4	21.5
20	17.0	20.3	17.6	21.7
21	14.4	21.8	21.8	21.5
22	16.2	22.8	21.8	22.3
23	19.1	18.3	21.8	21.2
24	17.6	19.8	21.4	21.5
25	28.8	15.4	20.9	22.5
26	19.2	16.9	20.3	22.3
27	19.0	17.4	19.5	22.5
28	21.4	23.9	20.4	21.4
29	16.1	15.6	20.4	21.4
30	19.4	22.5	20.2	20.8
31	16.7	24.0	20.7	22.1
32	18.8	14.9	22.0	22.2
33	19.2	22.0	17.6	22.9
34	18.7	13.2	20.8	22.6
35	15.3	15.1	21.2	21.7
36	19.3	13.7	20.7	21.5
37	17.4	26.8	16.4	22.0
38	15.2	20.4	17.6	21.9

(continued)

Item	A	B	C	D
39	14.9	16.4	21.0	22.8
40	21.5	17.2	19.6	22.4
41	19.6	19.2	21.8	22.6
42	19.2	16.4	19.7	22.1
43	20.3	20.8	18.4	22.3
44	19.1	17.1	18.3	21.1
45	16.9	23.8	22.5	22.0
46	13.9	16.2	21.8	22.6
47	13.1	20.0	24.2	22.4
48	15.3	17.0	17.8	22.6
49	20.7	17.4	16.8	22.2
50	20.0	15.4	20.0	22.1
51	18.7	16.7	17.3	22.2
52	20.0	26.1	19.6	21.8
53	18.7	18.3	20.3	22.4
54	16.7	15.0	15.5	20.8
55	15.3	20.5	20.4	22.7
56	12.3	15.3	22.3	22.9
57	18.2	20.6	19.9	23.4
58	18.5	22.2	17.7	22.1
59	16.2	18.6	19.0	22.1
60	17.8	14.1	17.7	22.3
61	17.6	23.9	20.9	22.4
62	16.5	22.8	19.8	21.6
63	18.2	16.0	21.7	21.5
64	14.9	16.8	18.1	21.9
65	20.7	20.3	19.2	20.9
66	18.1	17.6	18.4	22.2
67	14.8	24.8	19.9	21.6
68	16.4	19.3	21.1	22.8
69	15.9	20.3	20.9	21.6
70	17.7	19.0	21.4	22.8
71	20.1	20.8	21.3	22.6
72	19.0	20.8	21.3	23.0

(continued)

(continued from previous page)

Item	A	B	C	D
73	19.9	18.3	19.8	21.2
74	14.1	22.4	22.2	22.1
75	17.6	19.6	24.0	22.3
76	17.9	18.9	22.3	21.4
77	18.9	17.7	19.1	22.7
78	15.0	24.5	20.8	20.9
79	22.1	17.5	21.1	22.4
80	18.0	18.7	18.1	21.6
81	13.9	19.0	19.5	21.2
82	16.8	24.5	23.3	22.4
83	18.2	17.4	20.1	21.0
84	16.0	14.6	21.1	21.5
85	16.6	17.3	21.5	22.2
86	15.7	17.1	18.3	22.1
87	20.8	23.9	19.7	22.0
88	22.0	20.1	18.5	22.4
89	18.7	14.6	19.6	22.3
90	17.5	19.5	21.2	20.9
91	15.7	13.9	19.5	22.6
92	20.7	17.9	21.1	22.7
93	18.0	20.1	15.9	22.8
94	19.6	22.6	20.3	21.7
95	17.5	23.3	20.9	22.5
96	17.7	20.9	21.7	21.8
97	16.4	24.7	21.0	21.9
98	18.5	19.8	20.5	22.3
99	17.6	17.4	17.6	21.9
100	20.6	21.0	22.2	21.7

Analysis

What is the null hypothesis? In this case there are several null hypotheses, so state each one separately or else state the null hypothesis in a general way so as to include all possibilities. Is the null hypothesis supported to the confidence level required?

What location seems to be getting the best service on the basis of each of the measures? Is any significant difference found in the delivery times, and on what basis do you conclude that? Include a few charts in the report because this is a dispute among management, and therefore matters are not likely to be settled by pages of numbers.

Lessons Learned

You have now applied classical statistical tests to rich data sets. You also have selected suitable charts to portray the data and support the conclusion.

CASE 16: SEQUENTIAL ANALYSIS

Topic: Acceptance Testing

Occasionally, you may have to decide it is time to stop a test. Sequential testing supports an early decision on whether to accept a change. The method used here, while it may seem to be awfully simple, is just as rigorous as any other statistical method (Mood 1950).

The method to be applied here requires that the characteristics of the new distribution be known as well as the characteristics of the old distribution. The method can also be applied at the trial stage if the new distribution can be estimated. If new equipment is being evaluated to replace old equipment, the vendor of the new equipment may be able to give the analyst the expected lifetime or failure rate. (Note: If the vendor provides inflated, optimistic lifetimes for the new equipment, this method will punish the new equipment in the evaluation.)

This method does not require that the new distribution and the old distribution be of the same form. If both are normal distributions, that is fine. If one is a normal distribution and the other a Weibull bathtub distribution, that is fine, too. If the distributions are not well known but enough data are available to make a histogram, that is good enough. Scale the histogram so that the sum of all probabilities is 100 percent.

Here is the method:

1. Let the null hypothesis be that no difference exists between the old and the new distributions.
2. Pick a confidence level against false negatives.

3. Pick a confidence level against false positives.

    (To review, a *false negative* is a rejection of the null hypothesis when the conclusion should have been to accept the null hypothesis. A *false positive* is an acceptance of the null hypothesis when the conclusion should have been to reject the null hypothesis. The *null hypothesis* is that no difference exists between the two distributions.)

4. Compute two limits:
    - Limit A is the ratio of the false-positive confidence level to one minus the false-negative confidence level.
    - Limit B is the ratio of one minus the false-positive confidence level to the false-negative confidence level.

    For example, if the false-negative confidence level is 75 percent and the false-positive confidence level is 90 percent, Limit A is 90%/(1 – 75%), which equals 3.60, and Limit B is (1 – 90%)/75%, which equals 0.13. In general, Limit A will be greater than 1 and Limit B will be less than 1.

5. Gather the first sample. Evaluate the new distribution and the old distribution with this sample as the argument to the distribution function for each. Call these $V_{new,1}$ and $V_{old,1}$. Compute the ratio of $V_{new,1}$ to $V_{old,1}$, and call this $Ratio_1$.

6. Compare $Ratio_1$ with Limit A. If $Ratio_1$ is bigger than Limit A, *reject the null hypothesis.*

7. Compare $Ratio_1$ with Limit B. If $Ratio_1$ is smaller than Limit B, *accept the null hypothesis.*

8. If $Ratio_1$ is between the two, draw another sample. Perform the same evaluations to get to a new ratio, which will be called $Ratio_2$. Multiply $Ratio_1$ by $Ratio_2$, and call this $Product_2$. Compare $Product_2$ with the limits, applying the same tests and drawing the same conclusions.

9. Repeat as many times as necessary, multiplying all the ratios together each time and performing the limit tests on that product. Hence, for example, $Product_4 = Ratio_4 \times Ratio_3 \times Ratio_2 \times Ratio_1$.

    Compare $Product_4$ with Limit A. If $Product_4$ is bigger than Limit A, *reject the null hypothesis.*

    Compare $Product_4$ with Limit B. If $Product_4$ is smaller than Limit B, *accept the null hypothesis.*

10. In theory, the first time either Limit A or Limit B is crossed, the evaluation sequence can be terminated and the conclusion announced. Because, in practice, the two distributions are never known with high precision, it is prudent to gather a few more samples to confirm the result.

Work

1. Apply this method to the evaluation of battery lifetime for a certain handheld computer device. A vendor has come forward with a new battery that he claims has a 30 percent greater life. This is the same vendor who sold you the old ones, and he offers you the parameters for the Weibull bathtub curve lifetime distribution, saying his research laboratory has developed both the new and the old distributions on the basis of extensive field and laboratory testing. Given that many users have complained about the short life of the old batteries, and given that the price difference is small, you agree to conduct a trial test of the new batteries by putting them in 20 units and issuing them to regular users so that the tests will be representative.

2. The vendor asserts that the Weibull parameters for the old battery are 5 and 30, whereas the parameters for the new battery are 5 and 40. To see what this might look like, open a spreadsheet and evaluate the Weibull function for a range of values from 0 to 50. Work with the old battery data in one column and the new battery data in the next. Plot the results, showing both distributions on one chart, and include the chart in the report.

3. Start the trial. The first battery fails after 34 days. Apply the tests, using confidence limits of 80 percent and 90 percent for false-negative and false-positive tests. If the test is conclusive, declare victory.

    Applying the built-in Excel function for the old distribution, WEIBULL.DIST(34,5,30,false), gives 4.24 percent, and for the new distribution, WEIBULL.DIST(34,5,40,false), gives 4.19 percent. Because the two are quite close together, one would expect the test to be inconclusive.

4. If the test is inconclusive, wait for the next battery to fail and then apply the test to the product of the first two ratios as prescribed above.

5. Continue until one of the limits is crossed or until the trial population is exhausted.

6. Given that all of the 20 units are already in test, collect the battery life data as it comes in for all 20, and repeat the tests each time. Plot the products versus the failure-sequence number, and show the A and B limits on the plot. If the products get to be very large or very small, use some judgment about the plotting.

Data

Use this data set; it can also be found on the companion website, ache.org/books/6Sigma.

Sequence	Life	Sequence	Life
1	34.0	11	41.0
2	35.0	12	42.0
3	35.5	13	44.0
4	37.0	14	44.5
5	38.0	15	45.0
6	39.0	16	48.0
7	39.0	17	49.5
8	40.0	18	50.0
9	40.5	19	52.0
10	40.5	20	55.0

Analysis

The second parameter of the Weibull distribution is the lifetime parameter; 37 percent of all samples will have a lifetime greater than this parameter. For the new batteries, 37 percent can be expected to last to day 40. How does this compare with the actual results? For the old batteries, 37 percent can be expected to last to day 30. How does *this* compare with the actual results? On the basis of the actual lifetimes, would it be possible to choose between the two distributions? Suppose two of the batteries had been lost on day 35. Could this information be used in any way?

Lessons Learned

You have now applied both false-negative and false-positive confidence tests to sequential data.

CASE 17: RULE-INDUCED UPSETS

Topic: Management Effect on Service

This exercise will address local optimization versus global optimization. Management decides what is best for each patient while that patient is within the domain of that manager's unit and issues rules with the patient's best interest in mind. Each unit manager, however, has a focus of vision that is concentrated on that unit. Each manager cannot have the whole of the organization in mind at each moment.

Therefore, each unit manager makes rules that look a lot like local optimizations, even with the best interest of the patient in mind.

In this case, the surgery unit schedules its routine surgery cases in the morning; afterward, the patients are held in the surgery unit, where they can get the best care in case of some difficulty, until 11:30 a.m. At this point, those patients showing standard progress are moved to the postoperative patient care unit for bed rest and further care.

On a typical day, 10 to 12 patients make this move. Three orderlies and three elevators are available, so the patients are delivered in groups of three. The orderlies get back to the surgery unit and return with the next set of three patients in five minutes.

Logging the patient in to the postoperative unit, getting the patient moved into the assigned room, hooking up monitors, and so on take six minutes per patient. Two nurses are assigned to these tasks, and they work in parallel and draw on the patient care unit's aides and orderlies for help.

Work

1. Using a spreadsheet, tally the number of patients transferring into the postoperative pool at each minute. Tally the number moved out of the pool at each minute. Tally the pool count at each minute.
2. Calculate the average time, the 75 percent of population time, and the maximum time of patients' wait in the pool if 12 patients are being moved to postoperative care.
3. Analyze the data and create a chart or two to portray what is happening. Just float the cursor over the various chart-type icons and let Excel show you your data in a variety of presentations. Some will be more illuminating than others.

Data

No additional data are required for this case.

Analysis

Figuring that a long wait in the postoperative patient care unit pool to get to a bed is not the overall optimum situation for the patient, propose some different rules, equipment, or staffing that would likely improve this situation from the patient's point of view. Draft a recommendation, and apply a simple potential problem analysis to this recommendation. Reconsider the recommendation in light of the potential problem analysis and, if appropriate, modify the recommendation somewhat. Include this recommendation in the report.

Does the recommendation affect more than one unit? If so, what level in the organization does the recommendation have to reach?

Lessons Learned

You have now considered unit operating rules that are in the best interest of the patient from the point of view of that unit. You also have considered the rules' effect on the next unit and recommended a change that addresses the patient's best interest from a more global viewpoint.

CASE 18: IMPROVEMENT PROJECT

Topic: Snap-On Patient Monitors

A vendor proposes that the organization adopt the latest in snap-on patient monitors. This device fits over a thumb or big toe and is connected by wire to a computer and then to the computer network; it monitors pulse rate, blood pressure, and gross changes in blood sugar level. The computer associates each device with an assigned patient, and it knows if the device has slipped off or been moved in such a way as to lose its signals. The computer produces on-demand and on-trigger reports at the patient care unit station and can be accessed by authorized personnel using remote computer stations, two-way pagers, and other network devices.

The organization already uses some lower-functionality snap-on monitors on critical patients. However, due to the high cost of the older devices, they are not being used for general patients. The new devices are much cheaper and may be suitable for the general patient population.

The vendor has provided manufacturer's data supporting the following claims:

+ The failure rate of the new devices is very low—only one-thousandth of the failure rate of the older devices.
+ The software failure rate is less than once in any five-year period.

- Patients in a test program in another state did not complain of discomfort while wearing the devices.

Work

1. Design a trial program for the new device. Consider what populations to include and consider where those populations are in the building complex. Perform a potential problem analysis.
2. If the failure rate is truly low for the new device, and if the failure rate has been quite low for the older devices, on what basis will the trial be considered a success or failure? What quantitative analysis might you use? What data would you require for such quantitative analysis?
3. Make a recommendation to management.
4. Include your logic and some suitable charts in the report; maybe a process flow diagram would be useful, or maybe another type of diagram would be.

Data

No additional data are required for this case.

Analysis

One cost of using such devices on a regular basis is that small devices tend to get lost in the bedclothes and wander off in the pockets of discharged patients and visitors. Is this something to be considered in the design of the trial? If so, how would the trial take care of this?

If the trial is successful and the device is used very generally within the organization, what provisions should be made to deal with the exceptional patient who is allergic to the device or is bandaged in such a way that the device cannot be used?

Lessons Learned

You have now considered a technology upgrade from one highly reliable generation of computerized equipment to the next. You have designed a trial of the new generation principally on nonstatistical bases.

CASE 19: EVENT A

Topic: Bathroom Falls

A patient falls in the bathroom adjoining his room in the middle of the night. He suffers some minor injuries with no permanent consequences, but management, on consideration of the facts, decides the same fall might have been life-threatening if the circumstances had been different in exceedingly minor ways. Management declares this to be a significant event and wants a solution. A project manager and analyst are assigned.

On reviewing the records for the past three years, it comes to light that 14 falls have occurred in patients' bathrooms, but none have resulted in serious injury. Some facts about each fall are provided in the table in the "Data" section.

Each patient's bed has rails, a call button, and a step stool. Some patients are allowed to leave their bed to go to the bathroom on their own, and some are not. These latter patients are said to be "restricted to bed." The difficulty with figuring out what to do to reduce errors in this case is that it is the patient who is making the error. Training the patient does not seem very promising as a solution.

This appears to be an opportunity to apply poka-yoke in an effort to develop a system that is so easy to use that even untrained people—in this case, patients—will be more likely to do the right thing than the wrong thing.

How can the bathroom-fall hazard be mitigated? Is there something about access to the bathroom that might be mitigating? Something inside the bathroom that might be mitigating? Something about getting out of bed, short of restraining every patient, that might be mitigating? Is there something about the patient being on his or her own that might be mitigating?

Work

1. Examine the data for patterns. Are any patterns evident?
2. Perform a failure modes and effects analysis of the safety features already provided. Think poka-yoke.
3. Develop a trial program. Include a potential problem analysis. Include an analysis of the likely time duration of the trial.
4. Put the essentials in the report.

Data

Use the data given in the following table. Note that one fall may be counted in several different ways, so the totals exceed the number of individual falls.

Characteristic	Count of True	Count of False
Male	9	5
Elderly	10	4
First night in this bed and room	5	9
Restricted to bed	4	10
Used call button first	7	7
Had fallen before	1	13

Analysis

Does the proposed trial allow for a range of patient behaviors? Does the proposed trial rely on any change in patient behavior, and, if so, how will this be enforced? What sources of outside ideas should the analyst consider in seeking improvements to try?

Lessons Learned

You have just considered a very challenging matter: an error that is not being made by the system but is being allowed by the system, with the actual error being made by a patient who cannot be controlled by the system, short of using bed restraints. To solve this problem, you considered the poka-yoke approach to facilities design.

CASE 20: EVENT B

Topic: Pressure Ulcers

The organization provides bed care for periods of time typically running two to six weeks. Many patients have poor mobility. Some are subject to developing pressure ulcers (bed sores) if left by themselves in bed or in a wheelchair for extended periods of time. To reduce this likelihood, patients are turned in their beds twice each shift, and the patient may be awakened, if necessary, to do this. The patients are reseated in their wheelchairs during any extended chair time.

The turning is performed by orderlies. This work is done mid-shift and again near the end of the shift. These orderlies also have other duties assigned, some of which are highly variable in occurrence. At the end of each round, the orderlies sign a sheet indicating each patient who has been turned or who, for some reason, has not been turned.

The organization finds that the number of pressure ulcer cases, although low, is not as low as the incidence rate reported by comparable organizations. Pressure ulcers are a serious matter on their own, and the incidence of pressure ulcers may detract from the organization's hard-won reputation for giving good care. Management decides to take this matter seriously, even though this issue is not thought to be life-threatening. A project manager and analyst are assigned.

On review of the records, the project team decides that the existing policy is the right one and that something is going wrong in its implementation. What is needed is not a new policy but the same policy, and yet clearly a problem exists. What needs to be done?

Work

1. Conduct a failure modes and effects analysis.
2. Recommend a new trial of the present process.
3. Recommend appropriate trial measures.
4. Include a chart or two in the report.

Data

No additional data are required for this case.

Analysis

What long-term tracking do you recommend?

Lessons Learned

You have just applied the Six Sigma method to the rectification—rather than the improvement—of a process.

CASE 21: TRAFFIC ANALYSIS A

Topic: Traffic Analysis with No Queue

Consider a service offered to the public: for example, a nursing home. Demand varies from day to day. The length of stay varies from patient to patient. If the average demand and the average length of stay are known, then quite a lot can be estimated about the business. Note that no probabilities are required, only the averages. Recall that the same is true of the Poisson discrete distribution, where only the average value of the one parameter need be known. Here, the average value of each of two parameters need to be known. It's also necessary to know the fixed capacity of the system.

Erlang worked out the probability distribution for the likelihood that the next arriving customer would be blocked, which is to say that at the moment of arrival the system would already be running at capacity. Erlang also worked out the expected waiting time if arrivals in excess of capacity are kept in queue and then served when capacity opens up. Details are given in appendix A.

The Erlang B distribution applies when there is no queue. Blocked customers leave and do not come back. This applies to many situations in real life—situations where competition exists. The customer just goes to a competitor.

There are ways to manage the incoming flow of customers. One is to book appointments. Bear in mind, though, that appointments have to be scheduled with enough space between start times that the system will almost always be ready for the next customer on time. A scheduled service cannot run at theoretical capacity because some slack has to be planned in to cover variations in execution time. Also, if one customer drops out, there is no way to fill the slot and replace the revenue. Scheduling services adds to overhead, as does reminding people of an upcoming appointment.

Work

Consider a nursing home that competes with other nursing homes, all offering inpatient rehabilitation services. The nursing home wants to stay full, and yet the nursing home also wants to have a bed available every time a hospital calls to ask for a bed. On top of that, the demand varies from day to day. Each patient is independent of every other patient, and the actual stay times vary from very short to very long, with the average being seven days.

1. Assume that capacity is set at 30 beds.
2. Assume that the ownership, in order to maintain good relations with hospitals, wants to have at least one bed free 90 percent of the time, while at the same time maintaining occupancy as high as possible.
3. The Erlang B distribution applies. No queuing.
   Erlang B requires, as inputs, the capacity and the average traffic level. The average traffic level is the product of the arrivals per unit time and the average service time, which in this case is the patient-stay time.
4. Assume an average service time of seven days.
5. Consider a range of traffic levels. The traffic level is the product of the arrival rate and the stay duration, using the average value for each. This product is also equal to the average occupancy, so considering a range of traffic levels is the same as picking an average occupancy level, which is convenient for this analysis.
6. Erlang B says the likelihood that the next arrival will be blocked, because every bed is already occupied, is given by this ratio using standard spreadsheet functions:
   Erlang-B = Poisson(traffic, capacity, false) / Poisson(traffic, capacity, true), where the third parameter is true for cumulative and false for non-cumulative distributions. The use of the Poisson functions to calculate Erlang B and Erlang C is shown in appendix B.
7. It's more convenient to consider the likelihood that a bed is available than the likelihood all beds are taken, so calculate one minus blocking to determine availability.
8. Consider a range of average occupancies from 20 to 29 beds, keeping the capacity at 30 beds.
9. Plot.

Data

- Capacity: 30 beds
- Occupancy: range from 20 to 29 beds

Analysis

What do the results mean? What policy should management apply? What other parameters might management study before reaching a final policy? How could management test a new policy before making an irreversible decision? What measures should management apply to know whether the new policy is working? What exactly is management trading off here?

Lessons Learned

By applying the Erlang B statistical model to a practical case, you have come up with results to recommend a management policy.

CASE 22: TRAFFIC ANALYSIS B

Topic: Traffic Analysis with Queue

Consider a magnetic resonance imaging (MRI) center that accepts walk-in patients. The center has two MRI scanners. Consider that, while there are other MRI centers in the general area, experience shows that most patients will sit and wait their turn rather than go elsewhere. Even so, if many patients have to wait a long time, the center will get a bad reputation and will lose future business.

The Erlang C model applies because patients are willing to wait in queue.

In the past, the center had booked patients, rather than accepted walk-ins, and found that about 10 percent of booked patients did not show up or were disqualified, so revenue was about 10 percent lower than expected.

Work

Appendix B shows this formula is valid for Erlang C. This formula uses only the Poisson function that is available in all modern spreadsheet applications.

1. Use one hour as the time basis. Note the following:
   - The capacity of the system is 2 units.
   - The average service time is 20 minutes per patient. Convert this to 0.33 hours per patient to have consistent time units.
   - Examine a range of patient arrivals in one hour, from 0 to 6.

2. To proceed, calculate the traffic, which is the number of arrivals in the hour times the service time. For 0 to 6 arrivals in one hour, the traffic is 0×0.33, $1 \times 0.33, \ldots 6 \times 0.33$.
3. Calculate the slack in the system, which is the difference between the capacity and the average traffic, divided by the capacity. The slack for all six cases is $(2\text{-}0 \times 0.33)/2$, $(2\text{-}1 \times 0.33)/2$, $(2\text{-}2 \times 0.33)/2$, $(2\text{-}3 \times 0.33)/2$, $(2\text{-}4 \times 0.33)/2$, $(2\text{-}5 \times 0.33)/2$, and $(2\text{-}6 \times 0.33)/2$.
4. Calculate the likelihood that the next patient is blocked and has to wait in queue, using these simple calculations:
    P = Poisson(traffic, capacity, false), using the Excel Poisson function
    Pc = Poisson(traffic, capacity, true)
    Erlang-C = P / (slack × Pc + [1-slack] × P)
5. Now calculate the mean queuing time:
    Mean queuing time = Erlang-C × Service Time / (Capacity × slack)
    The mean queuing time goes up if blocking goes up or if the service time goes up. The queuing time goes down if the capacity goes up or if slack goes up.

Data

Use the following:
  - One hour as the time of interest
  - A capacity of two units
  - A service time of 20 minutes (convert to fraction of an hour)
  - A range of 0 to 6 arrivals in the time of interest

Analysis

Calculate blocking fraction and mean queuing time.
    Repeat using two hours and then four hours as the time of interest. Consider carefully which parameters have to be rescaled.
    One might expect the mean queue of more than two or four hours to be better (smaller) than for one hour. What do the calculations show?
    What happens if traffic exceeds capacity?
    Repeat at least one of the sets, changing the basis to no-queue. Use Erlang B to calculate blocking with no queue. How does no-queue blocking compare with with-queue blocking?

Evaluate the walk-in service as a business model in comparison with booked service, for which prior experience shows about 10 percent of the booked patients don't show up or are disqualified.

Consider what to do on the second shift, when the number of arrivals drops by 40 percent. Should one of the scanners be shut down to save operating and staff costs? At what fraction of day-shift traffic should the center shut down one scanner? Both scanners?

Lessons Learned

You have now applied the Erlang C statistical model to develop policies to recommend to management for the operation of the MRI center.

Bonus Cases

These cases are not part of the standard Six Sigma green belt and black belt training programs. They are included here for the enlightenment of our esteemed readers.

THE AMUSEMENT PARK WORKFLOW CASE SET

1. You are the manager of an amusement park. You have recently switched to all-you-can-ride admission pricing. Now you find that half of your customers want to ride your Really Big Roller Coaster and have to stand in line for an hour to get on the ride. While they are waiting, they are thinking vile things about you and, what is worse, they are not buying anything at the concession stands.

   Think up three things that you could do to alleviate the problem. Make arguments for each.

   Is this bunching, batching, pending, or queuing?

2. You find that at least one-quarter of those who ride the Really Big Roller Coaster get right back in line to ride it again. You would like to accommodate them because they are probably your best customers and are most likely to come to the park again soon, but you would like to make sure everyone who wants to ride the coaster gets at least one chance to do so.

   Think up three things you could do to ensure fair treatment for each customer who wants to ride the coaster.

3. Draw a time-value diagram from the point of view of the customer who is a coaster fan. Consider the admission fee payment a negative value. Use your

imagination for values to ascribe to riding the coaster, riding the carousel, and so on. Consider the purchase of a hot dog as a small positive value.

4. Draw a time-value diagram from the point of view of the owner of the amusement park. The admission fee has value to you. What else has value to you while the customer is in the park? Is keeping the customer in the park a positive or a negative to you?

5. Your customers drive to your facility and park their vehicles in your lot. On busy days, parking takes a while because of the crush of incoming cars in addition to the manner in which you want people to park. Because of this, several bottlenecks are possible in customer flow: getting parked, getting admitted, getting on the roller coaster, and getting out of the parking lot to go home.

   Because everything is under your control, you can force one of these to be the true bottleneck. Consider where you want the bottleneck to be. Defend your selection. How would you know whether your bottleneck management scheme is working?

6. To improve capacity, you consider breaking down the four-car roller coaster train into two two-car trains. You know the ride time will still be five minutes. The reloading time will be two minutes because this time is dictated by the slowest-moving passenger.

   Will making this change improve capacity? (Hint: Draw a time-value sketch for the four-car train, then draw additional traces for the two two-car trains. For what fraction of the time is each car in action?)

7. You have two more cars in storage. If you bring them out and put them in service, should it be as extra cars on one long train, as a separate two-car train, or as third cars on the existing two-car trains? Loading time will still be two minutes per train, regardless of train length. (Hint: Make more time-value sketches. Try a time-value sketch for the track.)

8. Your brother-in-law wants to open a soft drink concession stand just at the exit walkway from the Really Big Roller Coaster because he thinks this will catch a lot of customers who are excited from the ride. If he is right, about half of the coaster riders will stop at the new stand. Given that the passengers all come away from the coaster in a bunch, how many customers does the new stand have to serve, and how many minutes do they have to get the service done? Does it matter if the coaster is running one long train or two or three smaller trains? Is this bunching, batching, pending, or queuing?

9. Workers at the new concession stand can serve one customer every 30 seconds. People will not stand in line if the line already has more than three people in it. How many workers should the stand have? Why?

10. The stand can either have the worker handle payment, or it can have a separate cashier. If the workers only have to pour sodas, they can serve a customer every 20 seconds. The cashier can handle eight people per minute. Is one cashier enough? (Hint: Draw a time-value curve from the point of view of the customer. Considering queuing time to get the soft drink, work time to get the soft drink, queuing time to get to the cashier, and work time to pay the cashier.)

11. Cashiers are paid more than the workers who only dispense sodas. Customer service is more important than labor cost. Does that figure into the staffing strategy?

Selected Formulae

The following formulae have been selected for inclusion here because they underlie the statistical analysis currently provided by computer applications. These are presented for information only; familiarity with them is not required to follow the text or to apply the Six Sigma method.

The cumulative uniform distribution

$$F(x; a, b) = \int_a^b \frac{dx}{b - a}$$

The cumulative normal distribution

$$F(x; \mu, \sigma) = \int_{-\infty}^x \frac{1}{\sqrt{2\pi}\sigma} e^{-(x-\mu)^2/2\sigma^2} dx$$

The cumulative gamma distribution

$$F(x; \alpha, \beta) = \int_0^x \frac{1}{\alpha! \beta^{\alpha+1}} t^\alpha e^{-t/\beta} dt$$

The cumulative Poisson distribution

$$F(x'; \lambda) = \sum_0^{x'} \frac{e^{-x} \lambda^x}{x!}$$

The cumulative Student's t-distribution

$$F(t;n) = \int_{-\infty}^{t} \frac{\left(\frac{n-1}{2}\right)!}{\left(\frac{n-2}{2}\right)!\sqrt{\pi n}\left(1 + \frac{x^2}{n}\right)^{(n+1)/2}}\ dx$$

The Erlang B distribution

$$Erlang - B(E, m) = \frac{E^m/m!}{\sum_{i=0}^{m} E^i/i!}$$

The Erlang C distribution

$$Erlang - C(E, m; slack) = \frac{E^m/m!}{E^m/m! + slack * \sum_{k=0}^{m-1} E^k/k!}$$

Erlang Traffic Analysis

Capacity analysis—the trade-off between capital investment and various measures of service level—has been modeled successfully using only very simple inputs for about a hundred years. The hero in this development was Anger Erlang, who was employed by the Copenhagen telephone company in the early part of the twentieth century. The question before him was how to establish capacity requirements for telephone lines while attaining some level of customer satisfaction.

IT IS REMARKABLE that no breakthrough in the past century has displaced the Erlang statistical models, which are used today more to size telephone call centers than telephone lines and switches themselves. The general field of study is called *traffic engineering*, as the point of it all is to understand, manage, and design the system to carry the traffic while achieving management's goals for customer satisfaction.

Erlang derived the distribution of call arrivals on the basis of these points: that calls are independent of each other, that the duration of any call may be longer or shorter but with some mean value, that a call not served (blocked) may be dropped or kept in queue, and that only a small fraction of the total population of potential callers will seek service in any time period. From his theory, Erlang wrote down specific formulae for various matters, two of which are of interest in capacity planning and are discussed below.

First, consider the following:

- m, the number of beds
- Ts, the average bed-stay stated in days
- A, the average count of new arrivals each day, some of whom are admitted and some of whom are blocked
- E, the traffic level, which is A × Ts stated in bed days
- Slack, which is the fraction $(m - E)/m$; this is the average slack over a period of time

Here are the two Erlang formulae of interest for traffic analysis:

1. *Erlang B* is the likelihood that the next arrival is blocked and goes away, given the traffic and capacity.
2. *Erlang C* is the likelihood that the next arrival is blocked but put into a queue, given the traffic and capacity. In this case, arrivals already in queue are served before new arrivals are served.

Spreadsheets do not include the Erlang formulae. The purpose of this appendix is to restate the Erlang formulae in terms of Poisson distributions, because Poisson formulae are available in every modern spreadsheet.

ERLANG B

The Erlang B distribution (see Tanner 2000) is given by

$$EB(E, m) = \frac{E^m/m!}{\sum_{i=0}^{m} E^i/i!}$$

Recall that the Poisson distribution is given by

$$P(E, m) = \frac{e^{-E} E^m}{m!}$$

Because the Poisson distribution applies to discrete values of m, the cumulative of the Poisson distribution from zero to m is given by summing up from zero to m:

$$Pc(E, m) = e^{-E} \sum_{i=0}^{m} \frac{E^i}{i!}$$

Consider the ratio of the Poisson distribution function to the Poisson cumulative distribution function; thus,

$$\text{Ratio} = \frac{e^{-E} E^m/m!}{e^{-E} \sum_{i=0}^{m} E^i/i!}$$

Cancelling the exponential factor in the numerator and the denominator leaves

$$\text{Ratio} = \frac{E^m/m!}{\sum_{i=0}^{m} E^i/i!}$$

which, by inspection, is the same as the Erlang B formula. Therefore,

$$EB(E,m) = \frac{Poisson\ distribution(E,m)}{Cumulative\ Poisson\ distribution(E,m)}$$

The Poisson distributions are readily available in every modern spreadsheet program. In Excel, the function is POISSON(E, m, false) for the distribution and POISSON(E, m, true) for the cumulative distribution.

ERLANG C

The Erlang C distribution places blocked arrivals in a queue. When capacity opens up, the capacity is filled from the queue. Erlang C takes into account the slack in the system:

$$Slack = \frac{Capacity - traffic}{Capacity}$$

$$EC(E,m) = \frac{E^m/m!}{E^m/m! + slack * \sum_{k=0}^{m-1} E^k/k!}$$

Using the same notation as above for Poisson and cumulative Poisson, we get

$$EC(E,m) = \frac{P(E,m)}{P(E,m) + slack * Pc(E,m-1)}$$

Noting that the argument to the Pc term is $m - 1$ while the other terms have argument m, to proceed it is necessary to use the following:

$$Pc(E,m-1) = e^{-E} \sum_{i=0}^{m-1} E^i/i!$$

$$Pc(E,m-1) = Pc(E,m) - \frac{e^{-E}E^m}{m!}$$

The new term on the end is, by inspection, the Poisson distribution P(E, m), which allows all terms to have limits (E, m). Restating:

$$EC(E,m) = \frac{P(E,m)}{P(E,m) + slack * Pc(E,m) - slack * P(E,m)}$$

Regrouping in the denominator gives

$$EC(E,m) = \frac{P(E,m)}{(1 - slack) * P(E,m) + slack * Pc(E,m)}$$

So, the Erlang C distribution is now stated in terms of the Poisson distribution and the Poisson cumulative distribution, both of which are readily available in modern spreadsheets.

Recall that the Erlang B distribution allows no queue, while the Erlang C distribution does allow a queue. Suppose the slack is zero. In this case,

$$EC(E,m; slack = 0) = \frac{P(E,m)}{P(E,m)} = 1$$

In other words, the next arrival is always blocked. If there is no slack in the system, queuing doesn't help.

Suppose the slack is nearly unity, meaning that the facility is nearly empty. In this case,

$$EC(E,m; slack = 1) = \frac{P(E,m)}{Pc(E,m)} = EB(E,m)$$

Which is to say that the Erlang C distribution approaches the Erlang B distribution if the system has a lot of slack. This seems to make sense; if there is a lot of slack, there won't be any queue.

Annotated Bibliography

The literature on quality improvement in healthcare is extensive, and the literature on applied statistical methods is nearly as extensive. The following list includes sources cited in this book and other uncited sources that may be of interest to readers studying these fields. This is far from a complete listing, however, of all the sources that might be useful. The comments are offered with the intent to help the reader and are not meant as estimations of the works themselves. Indeed, these works are highly esteemed, or else they would not appear here.

Agency for Healthcare Research and Quality (AHRQ). 2016. "Never Events." Published July. http://psnet.ahrq.gov/primers/primer/3/never-events.

> Updated from time to time, this is a list of medical events that put patients at risk and that should never happen. The first list in this series was put forward in 2011 by Dr. Ken Kizer, formerly CEO of the National Quality Forum. Eliminating the events on the list should be a key goal of every healthcare organization.

Aguayo, R. 1990. *Dr. Deming, the American Who Taught the Japanese About Quality.* Secaucus, NJ: Lyle Stuart.

> This book is filled with case studies offered by a consultant who worked with Deming. Despite the title, the book is not a biography.

ASQ Quality Press. 2013. *TQM: Introduction to and Overview of Total Quality Management.* Milwaukee, WI: ASQ Quality Press.

> This book is a collection of helpful articles. TQM features continuous improvement and all-hands involvement.

Associated Press. 2015. "Social Security Records Show 6.5 Million Are 112-Years-Old, but That Can't Be Right." AL.com. Published March 14. www.al.com/news/index.ssf/2015/03/social_security_records_show_6.html.

> The Social Security database is about as simple as any database can be. Even so, it has a lot of problems with data entry and fraud.

Barry, R. 2003. *Nan: A Six Sigma Mystery.* Milwaukee, WI: ASQ Quality Press.

> New head nurse and Six Sigma Black Belt Nan solves a mystery and teaches her staff Six Sigma principles along the way. By the end of the book, Nan's department loves her and everybody else is mad at her.

————. 2004. *Nan's Arsonist: A Six Sigma Mystery.* Milwaukee, WI: ASQ Quality Press.

> Nan solves another mystery, continues to teach Six Sigma principles, and learns to get along with the other departments.

————. Forthcoming. *Nan Takes Home: A Six Sigma Mystery.* Milwaukee, WI: ASQ Quality Press.

> Nan solves a mystery, continues to teach Six Sigma principles, and finally learns to get along with her boss.

Barry, R., and A. Smith. 2005. *The Manager's Guide to Six Sigma in Healthcare.* Milwaukee, WI: ASQ Quality Press.

> This is an introduction to Six Sigma with short chapters on a wide range of subjects.

Bennett, J. 2012. "Top Ten Medical Uses of the iPhone." Posted December 14. http://internetmedicine.com/2012/12/14/top-ten-medical-uses-of-the-iphone/.

> This article lists many more than ten attachments that turn an iPhone or smartphone into a medical device such as an otoscope, ultrasound, or EKG.

Breyfogle, F. W. III. 1999. *Implementing Six Sigma: Smarter Solutions Using Statistical Methods.* New York: Wiley.

> This book is a thorough presentation of Six Sigma factory applications for an engineering audience and includes equations, tables, and drills. The text brings Henry James to mind.

Breyfogle, F. W. III, J. M. Cupello, and B. Meadows. 2000. *Managing Six Sigma: A Practical Guide to Understanding, Assessing, and Implementing the Strategy That Yields Bottom-Line Success.* New York: Wiley.

> This book is intended for managers and is nearly equation-free. It describes why and how to apply Six Sigma and includes a few case studies. It is a well-written text with the intent to cover service industries as well as manufacturing industries, but the service industries are limited to transaction processors.

Cassin, B. R., and P. R. Barach. 2012. "Making Sense of Root Cause Analysis Investigations of Surgery-Related Adverse Events." *Surgical Clinics of North America* 92 (1): 101–15.

This article criticizes root case analysis for being too mechanical and not paying enough consideration to human and organizational factors.

Chassin, M. R., and J. M. Loeb. 2013. "High-Reliability Health Care: Getting There from Here." *Milbank Quarterly* 91 (3): 459–90. www.jointcommission.org /assets/1/6/Chassin_and_Loeb_0913_final.pdf.

The article makes the argument that high-reliability status for healthcare organizations is a noble goal but one that is presently out of reach. For the next several years, healthcare should concentrate on process improvement with means such as Six Sigma, Lean, and change management.

Chicago Historical Society and the Trustees of Northwestern University. 1996. "The Great Conflagration." Accessed December 2, 2016. www.chicagohs.org/fire /conflag/.

This site includes narration of the Chicago fire by witnesses, plus extracts from the *Chicago Tribune*, whose brand-new and supposedly fireproof office tower in the center of the city burned to the ground. The records show the fire started in or near the O'Leary barn. The cow is folklore, but somebody must have kicked over the lantern, wouldn't you agree?

Crosby, P. 1979. *Quality Is Free*. New York: McGraw-Hill.

This book reawakened American industry to quality as a business interest. It's free! Many found it to be so. Six Sigma derives directly from Crosby's work, which focuses on getting rid of errors, albeit with less specificity than Six Sigma applies. Crosby declared that quality is the satisfaction of requirements and nothing else, and this is an important point in the development of Six Sigma. Crosby has also said that Six Sigma is not aggressive enough, and that the only right answer is no error at all.

DeVita, M., J. Schaefer, T. Dongilli, H. Wang, and J. Lutz. 2004. *Improving Medical Crisis Team Performance Using a Computerized Human Patient Simulator*. University of Pittsburgh Winter Institute for Simulation Education and Research. Accessed December 2, 2016. www.wiser.pitt.edu/sites/wiser/news/2004/03/media /imms_devita_poster.pdf.

This is a good example of training ad hoc teams by drills using simulated patient events—in this case, cross-training so that trainees learn the duties of several positions.

Emerson, R. W. 1860. "Culture." In *The Conduct of Life*, ch. IV. Revised 1876.

A fuller citation is more amusing, not something one seeks in Emerson as a rule: "Colonel, that none but a poltroon will boast that he never was afraid. A great part of courage is the courage of having done the thing before."

Gaba, D. M., K. J. Fish, and S. K. Howard. 1994. *Crisis Management in Anesthesiology*. Philadelphia, PA: Harcourt.

> Dr. Gaba is a pioneer in reducing error in anesthesiology, and in this book he catalogs special events and how to handle them. See also www.med.stanford.edu/profiles/david-gaba?tab=publications.

Gawande, A. 2009. *The Checklist Manifesto*. New York: Metropolitan Books.

> Dr. Gawande learns that the hyperspecialization of modern medicine requires that the work and communications be organized in ways that are entirely new to medicine but well known in other fields. A gifted writer, Dr. Gawande is a doctor with a mind full of wonder.

———. 2004. Lecture as part of book tour, Carnegie Music Hall, Pittsburgh, PA, March 9.

> See also www.atulgawande.com for publications. Dr. Gawande writes for *The New Yorker* and has published four books, all of which are good. In particular, see *The Checklist Manifesto*.

Gilbreth, F. B. 1912. *Primer of Scientific Management*. New York: D. Van Nostrand Company.

> Frank and his wife Lillian were efficiency experts of the old school. They loved stopwatches, shot miles of film of workers, and broke tasks down to the specific arm movements. Their professional work is cited at www.accel-team.com/scientific/scientific_03.html. For a delightful story of how they applied their efficiency theories at home with their 12 children, see Gilbreth, F. Jr., and E. Gilbreth. 1950. *Cheaper by the Dozen*. Chicago: Dramatic Publishing Company. Not much about their professional work is discussed there, but then if you've seen one stopwatch, you've seen them all. A movie of the story (MGM 1950) is reviewed online at www.rinkworks.com/movies/m/cheaper.by.the.dozen.1950.shtml.

Goldratt, E. M., and J. Cox. 1984. *The Goal: Excellence in Manufacturing*. New York: North River Press.

> Everyone should write like this! It's a novel; the hero discovers Goldratt's principles as he struggles with factory problems familiar to any industrialist. There are no equations. Goldratt is a mathematician who elaborated the mathematical principles underlying the Japanese Kanban/low-inventory system, which is the foundation of the workflow analysis used in this book. This classic first edition is highly recommended for all audiences and all managers, particularly in healthcare.

Google. 2016. "Google Flu Trends." Updated March 1. http://google.about.com /od/experimentalgoogletools/qt/GoogleFluTrends.htm.

> Google studied queries and found a concurrent indicator of flu outbreaks by geography, yielding better results than government reports, which have a two-week lag. This is called *now-casting* and is quite controversial because there is no mechanism to connect the particulars of the query to flu. Still, it seems to work. Google presently restricts access to the tool to academic researchers.

Gribbin, A. 2002. "Hospital Health Hazard." *Washington Times.* Published February 10. Retrieved from www.highbeam.com/doc/1G1-83549993.html.

> Gribbin cites reports from the Occupational Safety and Health Administration and other federal agencies on the incidence of assaults in emergency departments, psychiatric hospitals, and elsewhere. In the 1980s, at least 106 healthcare workers died as the result of assault.

Healthcare Finance Staff. 2013. "Medicare, Medicaid Error Estimates Grew in 2013." *Healthcare Finance News.* Published December 27. www.healthcarefinance news.com/news/medicare-medicaid-error-estimates-grew-2013.

Institute of Medicine (IOM). 2001. *Crossing the Quality Chasm: The IOM Health Care Quality Initiative.* Washington, DC: US National Academy of Sciences, Engineering, and Medicine, Health and Medicine Division.

Joint Commission. 2016a. *Sentinel Event Policy and Procedures.* Published January 6. www.jointcommission.org/sentinel_event_policy_and_procedures/.

> This is an analysis of life-threatening events and a workbook for dealing with such incidents.

————. 2016b. *2016 Hospital Accreditation Standards.* Published January. www .jcrinc.com/2016-hospital-accreditation-standards/.

> Following Joint Commission standards is voluntary. Standards are issued for hospitals and a variety of other healthcare organizations.

Juran, J. M. 1995. *Managerial Breakthrough*, revised ed. New York: McGraw-Hill.

> This is one of the very best books for management on both the why and the how of quality as a competitive weapon. Juran is one of the founders of the modern quality movement and should be read for that reason alone. It is also a good book that gets right to the point, and it has been written for managers, not statisticians.

Kaplan, R. 2010. "Conceptual Foundations of the Balanced Scorecard." Harvard Business School Working Paper 10-074.

Robert Kaplan and David Norton published the *Balanced Scorecard* in 1992. This paper is an evaluation after several years of experience.

Kazandjian, V. A. (ed.). 1997. *The Effectiveness of CQI in Health Care.* Milwaukee, WI: ASQ Quality Press.
   This is a compendium of reports on healthcare quality projects from the expected places (Holland, Japan, and others) and from some surprising ones (Niger).

Kennard, J. 2016. "Ultrasound Treatment for Prostate Cancer." *Verywell.* Published May 18. www.verywell.com/ultrasound-treatment-for-prostate-cancer-2329028.
   HIFU is a noninvasive procedure to treat certain cases of prostate cancer by focusing several ultrasound beams on target cells. Computer controlled, HIFU achieves results beyond what a human can.

Kirk, R. 1997. *Managing Outcomes, Process, and Cost in a Managed Care Environment.* Gaithersburg, MD: Aspen.
   This is a how-to book on applying quality programs in the healthcare arena with forms, charts, and step-by-step instructions. Witty and easy to follow, this book is closer to total quality management than to other regimens.

Kulbatski, I. 2016. "Novel 3-D 'Smart' Sutures for Wireless Collection of Biological Data." *medGadget.* Published July 18. www.medgadget.com/2016/07/novel-3-dimensional-smart-sutures-wireless-collection-biological-data.html.
   This article discusses sutures that are enhanced with tiny biological sensors plus computers and Bluetooth networking. Because the sutures can be placed well inside the skin, smart sutures have an advantage over surface-mounted smart Band-Aids.

Leveson, N. G. 1995. *Safeware, System Safety and Computers.* New York: Addison Wesley.
   This book deals with ultrareliable software system design for NASA and reports on safety event analysis in aviation and other industries. Timeless. Thoughtful. Incomparable.

Lieber, J. B. 2015. *Killer Care: How Medical Error Became America's Third Largest Cause of Death, and What Can Be Done About It.* New York: OR Books.
   This book is written by an attorney who has an interesting perspective. It includes lots of helpful information and anecdotes. Some good ideas, too.

Luthra, S. 2016. "Doctors Are Overloaded with Electronic Alerts, and That's Bad for Patients." *Washington Post.* Published June 13. www.washingtonpost.com/national

/health-science/doctors-are-overloaded-with-electronic-alerts-and-thats-bad-for-pati
ents/2016/06/10/0cae6b4a-20fa-11e6-9e7f-57890b612299_story.html.

Too many computers, meaning well, send bulletins about each patient at each little event. The results? Overload. Blizzard. Petulance. What to do? Ms. Luthra should perhaps read our book.

Magee, J. M. 2015. "The Four Causes." *Aquinas Online.* Updated March 20. www
.aquinasonline.com/Topics/4causes.html.

Mango, P. D., and L. A. Shapiro. 2001. "Hospitals Get Serious About Operations."
McKinsey Quarterly 2: 74–85.

This article is written by a business consulting firm, not medical researchers, for a business audience.

McFarland, M. 2012. "The Human Cost of Computer Errors." Markkula Center for Applied Ethics, Santa Clara University. Published June 1. www.scu.edu/ethics
/focus-areas/internet-ethics/resources/the-human-cost-of-computer-errors/.

This article discusses the implications of error in important databases, such as credit reports (agencies make 100,000 corrections per year after complaints), FBI identification records (where only 25 percent of submissions are correct and complete), and so on. Note that these are much simpler databases than patient records.

McKee, M. K., with S. Swanson. 2002. "Intensive Care." *Information Week,* June 17, 20.

The article features Xerox as a company focusing on computerization of physicians' orders as a way to serve mankind and shareholders at the same time.

McLaughlin, C. P., and A. D. Kaluzny. 1994. *Continuous Quality Improvement in Health Care.* Gaithersburg, MD: Aspen.

This book is an introduction to quality principles from Deming, Crosby, Juran, and others. Case studies in healthcare are contributed by various authors. The test at the end of the book blends total quality management and continuous quality improvement.

Meisenheimer, C. G. 1997. *Improving Quality: A Guide to Effective Programs,* 2nd ed. Gaithersburg, MD: Aspen.

This book is an excellent history of quality initiatives in healthcare since 1900! It includes the standards of The Joint Commission and compares quality assurance with quality improvement.

Montgomery, D. C. 1991. *Introduction to Statistical Quality Control,* 2nd ed. New York: Wiley.

This is the standard engineering textbook on applied statistics. It is a technique and applications text, not a guide to quality management, but it is an excellent technical reference book.

Mood, A. M. 1950. *Introduction to the Theory of Statistics*. New York: McGraw-Hill.
This graduate-level statistics text was written before computers were common, back when it was necessary to think things through.

Morse, S. 2016. "Analyze This: Health Systems, Health Plans Get to the Core of Big Data." *Healthcare Finance*. Published May 11. www.healthcarefinancenews.com/news/analyze-health-systems-health-plans-get-core-big-data.
Searching through big patient record sets is only meaningful if the data that were entered are sound.

Murphy, E. A. 1949. Air Force Captain.
Namesake of Murphy's Law: Anything that can go wrong, will go wrong. Or, Nature sides with the hidden flaw. Or, the perversity of inanimate things.

National Institute of Standards and Technology (NIST). 2016. "Baldrige Performance Excellence Program." Accessed September 22. www.nist.gov/baldrige.
Formerly known as the Bureau of Standards, NIST issues criteria for the Baldrige Awards in healthcare and other industries. The Baldrige criteria vary slightly from year to year. The website provides the current criteria and a wealth of information about the healthcare program.

———. 2001. *Malcolm Baldrige Criteria for Health Care 2001*. Washington, DC: National Institute of Standards and Technology.
Learn more about NIST and the Baldrige program at www.nist.gov.

Nerny, C. 2015. "Ridding EHRs of Dangerous, Often Undetectable, Bad Data." *Healthcare IT News*. Published March 13. www.healthcareitnews.com/news/ridding-ehrs-dangerous-often-undetectable-bad-data.
"Bad data in the system limits the effectiveness of clinical communications and decision support." Amen.

Occupational Safety and Health Administration (OSHA). 2013. *Caring for Our Caregivers: Facts About Hospital Worker Safety*. Published September. www.osha.gov/dsg/hospitals/documents/1.2_Factbook_508.pdf.
In 2011, US hospitals recorded 6.8 work-related injuries and illnesses for every 100 full-time employees, nearly double the rate for all private industry. From 2003 to 2011, 76 fatalities resulted from violence.

Paparrizos, J., R. W. White, and E. Horvitz. 2016. "Screening for Pancreatic Adenocarcinoma Using Signals from Web Search Logs: Feasibility Study and Results." *Journal of Oncology Practice* 12 (8): 737–44.

This study looked at Microsoft Bing search engine queries; results showed that query patterns can identify pancreatic cancer patients quite early.

Parkinson, C. N. 1957. *Parkinson's Law*. Boston: Houghton Mifflin.

This book is hilarious research into bureaucratic wonts.

Patient Advocators Organization (PAO). 2017. "About Patient Advocates." Accessed January 20. www.patientadvocators.com.

While other organizations specialize in billing, PAO focuses on the patient experience, providing advice on getting a second opinion, accompanying someone to the doctor's office, monitoring hospital stays, organizing records, and analyzing bills.

Peter, L. J. 1979. *Peter's People and Their Marvelous Ideas*. New York: William Morrow.

This book includes not only the Peter Principle but scores of other "laws" and aphorisms that are as delightful as they are instructive. See also *The Peter Pyramid*, published in 1986.

Peters, T. J., and R. H. Waterman Jr. 1982. *In Search of Excellence*. New York: Harper & Row.

This book is the timely story of a collection of companies that were trying hard to do things right. It is the first in a series of such books by Peters, who makes the point that the "excellent companies," by their very striving, ignite a passion in their employees.

PIAA. 2017. "Data Sharing Project." Accessed January 23. https://piaa.us/wcm/Data_Sharing_Project/wcm/_Data_Sharing_Project/What_is_the_DSP.aspx?hkey=e5c14723-790e-4326-8a44-ceea2455cc63.

Available to the public, this medical malpractice database helps identify markers that might have made a difference in various troubling cases.

Press Ganey. 2017. "National Database of Nursing Quality Indicators (NDNQI)." Accessed January 23. www.pressganey.com/solutions/clinical-quality/nursing-quality.

Press Ganey is the dominant company in patient satisfaction questionnaires and follow-up, used by practically every hospital and many other healthcare providers. The NDNQI is the national database of nursing quality indicators.

Reason, J. 1990. *Human Error*. New York: Cambridge University Press.

> This book is cited repeatedly in the famous 1999 Institute of Medicine report "To Err Is Human: Building a Safer Health System," available at www.national academies.org/hmd/. Mr. Reason has written other books in the series, but this one is the best known.

ResearchGate. 2017. "Advance Your Research." Accessed January 23. www .ResearchGate.net.

> ResearchGate provides a downloadable report on the application of the Balanced Scorecard methodology to several hospitals.

Rhythm Diagnostic Systems. 2017. "Our Solutions." Accessed January 23. www .rhythmdiagnosticsystems.com/solutions/.

> Rhythm Diagnostic Systems is a leading company in the smart Band-Aid field.

Rosander, A. C. 1991. *Deming's 14 Points Applied to Services*. New York: Marcel Dekker.

> The book contains case studies of Deming applications, though not in healthcare.

Ryan, M. J. R., and W. P. Thompson. 1998. *CQI and the Renovation of an American Health Care System*. Milwaukee, WI: ASQ Quality Press.

> This is the story of one large health system's progress through applied continuous quality improvement. It also deals with intangibles and the challenges of managing a multisite group.

Shingo, S. 1981. *Study of the Toyota Manufacturing System*. Tokyo, Japan: Japanese Management Association.

> This book contains case studies for rapid setup, small batch, Kanban manufacturing, and the progressive substitution of machine effort for human effort; poka-yoke is the recurring error-reduction method. This is the real source for the post–World War II Japanese revival of manufacturing.

Slabodkin, G. 2016. "Feds Take Another Step Toward Approving Wireless Body Sensors." *Health Data Management*. Published June 21. www.healthdatamanagement .com/news/feds-takes-another-step-toward-approving-wireless-body-sensors.

> The United States is the first country to allocate spectrum for "medical body area networks." The Federal Communications Commission allocated 40 megahertz of spectrum in the 2360 to 2400 MHz band, which is near the popular WiFi 2400 MHz frequency.

Smith, A., R. Barry, and C. Brubaker. 2007. *Going Lean: Busting Barriers to Patient Flow.* Chicago: Health Administration Press.

This book puts emphasis on well-managed workflow with a large collection of success stories from across the country.

Solet, J. M., and P. R. Barach. 2012. "Managing Alarm Fatigue in Cardiac Care." *Progress in Pediatric Cardiology* 33 (1): 85–90.

This article discusses false alarms, too many alarms, lack of prioritization, and the number of deaths estimated to have been caused by these problems.

StatSoft. 2013. *Electronic Statistics Textbook.* Tulsa, OK: StatSoft. www.statsoft.com /textbook/stathome.html.

StatSoft, a commercial provider of statistical software, offers a very good introductory-level online software textbook.

Student (Gosset, W. S.). 1908. "The Probable Error of a Mean." *Biometrika* 6 (1): 1–25.

Gosset was a self-taught amateur statistician who created the Student t-test, among other feats. Gossett was a brewer for Guinness.

Taguchi, G. 1978. "Off-line and On-line Quality Control Systems." In *Proceedings of the International Conference on Quality Control,* B4-1–B4-5. Tokyo, Japan: International Conference on Quality Control.

Taguchi introduced the important idea of uniform satisfaction of requirements, which is key to Six Sigma.

Tanner, M. 2000. "The Erlang-C Formula." www.mitan.co.uk/erlang/elgcmath.htm. On this web page, Tanner develops the application of the Erlang C formula; other pages on the site cover Erlang B. There are other websites that apply the Erlang formulae, and some even do the calculation online. The method of our present book is to express Erlang B and C in terms of Poisson distributions so that standard spreadsheets can perform the calculations. Erlang C is particularly popular these days to model call centers, which continue the telephone heritage going right back to Erlang. The equations work for any finite-capacity system, though, not just telephones.

Taylor, F. W. 1911. *The Principles of Scientific Management.* New York: Harper.

This is the original efficiency-by-stopwatch book, although most of Taylor's gains in productivity were achieved through improved ergonomics.

Tucker, A. L., and S. J. Spear. 2006. "Operational Failures and Interruptions in Hospital Nursing." *Health Services Research* 41 (3 Pt. 1): 643–62.
    Business professor Tucker has pioneered the study of interruptions in nursing tasks and duties.

US Food and Drug Administration (FDA). 2016. "FDA Approves First MRI-Guided Focused Ultrasound Device to Treat Essential Tremor." Published July 16. www.fda .gov/NewsEvents/Newsroom/PressAnnouncements/ucm510595.htm.
    This is an application of computer-generated ultrasound, like HIFU, applied to ablate brain tissue to treat essential tremor. The procedure was FDA approved in 2016.

US Navy Commander (initials CGD). 1974. Personal communication with the author (Barry).

Walton, M. 1990. *Deming Management at Work.* Boston: Perigee Books.
    This book contains case studies of the Deming method, including a case study of the Hospital Corporation of America. Others range from the Ford Motor Company to the US Navy. Perhaps the most interesting case is Tri-Cities, Tennessee, where a whole region tried to apply Deming's principles to every company in the area.

———. 1986. *The Deming Management Method.* Boston: Perigee Books.
    Walton worked with Deming and provides a readable book with many Deming anecdotes.

Weick, K. E., and K. M. Sutcliffe. 2001. *Managing the Unexpected: Resilient Performance in an Age of Uncertainty.* San Francisco: Jossey-Bass.
    This is the seminal work in the study of High-Reliability Organizations—organizations that have learned to deal with inherent risk through a specific management culture that can, perhaps, be applied to healthcare organizations. A second edition of the book was published in 2007. See also www .high-reliability.org.

Xenex. 2017. "Solutions." Accessed January 23. www.xenex.com/our-solutions.
    The Xenex robot conducts full-spectrum UV germ zapping when placed in a hospital room after a patient is discharged. It is important to the fight against infection.

Glossary

This glossary includes specialized words from the text, plus standard terminology from the field.

Topic	Discussion
ANOVA	Analysis of variance.
A priori, a posteriori	Before the fact, after the fact; sometimes written with hyphens or italicized for clarity.
Average	The arithmetic sum of the values in a set divided by the number of members of that set.
Baldrige Award	Federal quality award named for the Honorable Malcolm Baldrige, a former US Secretary of Commerce.
Bathtub curve	A distribution that is high at both ends and low in the middle, faintly reminiscent of the shape of a bathtub.
Chi-square distribution	The distribution of a variate defined as the square of the ratio of (the difference between a sample value and the sample average value) to the standard deviation of the underlying distribution.
Clinical pathways	A systematic method for studying workflow in a healthcare organization.
Confidence interval	An interval in which, to a specified level of confidence, a parameter being estimated lies.
Confidence level	An a priori probability to be associated with a confidence interval.

Control chart	A chart that portrays sample values plotted against a sample number or time.
Degrees of freedom	The number of samples available.
Erlang B	The probability of the next arrival being blocked, or refused service, in a finite capacity system with no ability to hold arrivals in queue.
Erlang C	The probability of the next arrival being blocked, or refused service, in a finite capacity system that can hold all arrivals in a queue.
Expectation	The probability of a specified outcome.
False negative	The finding of a negative outcome in a trial that is false; finding false when the outcome should have been true.
False positive	The finding of a positive outcome in a trial that is false; finding true when the outcome should have been false.
F distribution	The distribution of a variate that is the ratio of two variables independently distributed by chi-square distributions.
High-Reliability Organization	An organization in a hazardous industry able to achieve its goals, consistently over time, while dealing with uncertainty, change, and external events.
Histogram	A chart showing the frequency of occurrence of each of several outcomes.
ISO, ISO 9000	International Organization for Standardization (or ISO) standards in the 9000 group, which have to do with quality assurance; the ISO issues standards on many topics.
The Joint Commission	A nonprofit organization that certifies and accredits more than 20,000 US healthcare programs and organizations.
Kanban	Production on demand, particularly in small batches; the name is the anglicized form of the Japanese word for "punch card."

Keisen, Kaizen	Anglicized version of the Japanese term for "continuous improvement"; many English spellings are used.
Law, in statistics	A rule governing the behavior of a variate.
Likelihood	Probability of a specific outcome.
Mean	The numerical average of all results, weighted by the frequency of occurrence.
Murphy's Law	Anything that can go wrong will go wrong. Or, nature sides with the hidden flaw.
Normal distribution	The commonly occurring bell-shaped distribution, the equation for which uses the negative exponential of a squared variate; elaborated on by Gauss. The term "normal" is applied because the distribution appears very often and always appears when the matter being observed is the result of several operations.
Pareto Principle	An 80/20 rule of thumb; for example, 80 percent of sales come from 20 percent of the customer base.
Parkinson's Law	Work expands to fill the time available; there are many variations on this law.
Peter Principle	Managers are promoted to their level of incompetence, which is defined as one level beyond their level of competence.
Poka-yoke	The systematic design of work tasks so that the worker finds it easier to do the right thing than the wrong thing, rendering any error immediately obvious, and providing opportunity for errors to be rectified on the spot. The words mean "prevention of inadvertent error."
Population	The count of, or the definition of, a discrete group; for example, the population of patients, X-ray files, or magnetic resonance imaging machines.

Probability	The ratio of the number of occurrences of a specific outcome to the number of all possible outcomes; a probability is always between zero and one. For example: The probability of drawing the jack of clubs from a pack is 1 in 52; the probability of drawing a jack of any suit is 4 in 52; the probability of drawing a club of any rank is 13 in 52; the probability of the drawn card being a jack, given that it is a club, is 1 in 13; the probability of the drawn card being a club, given that it is a jack, is 1 in 4; the probability of drawing the same card twice in a row is 1 in 52.
Process control limits	Lines drawn for convenience on a control chart, displaced three standard deviations from the average value. These are convenient because data points will fall outside these lines only about once in 1,000 times if the process is following a normal distribution with fixed parameters; any point outside the control limits is unlikely and therefore suspect.
Quality assurance	The administration of the production process with a view toward producing consistent outcomes.
Regression	Fitting a selected equation to data samples; for example, linear regression fits a straight line.
Residual	The square of the difference in values between a sample and its expected value calculated from some equation, usually an equation fitted to the data samples.
Rich data set	A data set with a large number of data points, usually at least 50.
Scientific management	The study of work, tasks, human behavior in the workplace, the flow of work, and related matters, with emphasis on quantification.
Sigma (Σ, σ)	Greek letter that is commonly used, in lowercase, to represent the standard deviation.

Significance	A measure of an unlikely outcome; an outcome that is significant at the 0.05 level would be expected to happen only 5 percent of the time; the significance level and the confidence level together add up to 100 percent.
Six Sigma	A management method to reduce errors to the specific level of 3.4 errors per million in practical organizations.
Sparse data set	A data set with only a few data points, usually fewer than 25.
Standard deviation	The square root of the variance.
Student's t-distribution	The distribution of a variate that is the ratio of a normally distributed variate to the square root of a variate independently distributed by the chi-square law; this is valuable because a priori knowledge of the standard deviation of the underlying distribution is not needed; "Student" was the nom de plume of the discoverer of this distribution, William Sealy Gosset.
System limits	Lines on a control chart displaced six standard deviations away from the average value; these lines will be exceeded by normal fluctuations only very rarely, so the organization can plan its work on the idea that the system limits will not be exceeded in a particular work unit.
Underlying distribution	Data samples are acquired and analyzed to estimate the parameters of the distribution from which the samples arose; this distribution is called the underlying distribution.
Uniform distribution	A distribution for which all outcomes are equally likely, as is found when flipping a coin or drawing a card from a deck.
Variance	The sum of the squares of the differences among sample values and the average value; this definition applies to all distributions.

Variate	A mathematical entity that takes on values according to a distribution, rule, or law.
Weibull distribution	A distribution, attributed to Weibull, that is often used to model lifetime behavior, including bathtub-profile behavior and exponential lifetimes.
Yield	The ratio of desired outcomes to all outcomes.

Index

About the Authors

This second edition has been updated by the three authors of the first edition.

Robert Barry, PE, PhD, is CEO of Balester Group LLC; an adjunct professor for the University of Pittsburgh; a certified Six Sigma master black belt; and a management consultant specializing in systems of extremely high reliability, with clients ranging from hospitals and utilities to the Alaska Pipeline. Dr. Barry formerly was managing principal for Caldwell Butler & Associates LLC. He received a bachelor's degree from Iowa State University, earned his master's and doctoral degrees from the University of Pittsburgh, and completed executive management programs at the Harvard Business School and Harvard Law School. Dr. Barry holds 11 US patents and has published widely on technical and management topics. He has held international executive positions for Westinghouse Energy Systems, has served on the faculty of The Pennsylvania State University, and is active in nonprofit organizations promoting the education and employment of people with severe physical and sensory handicaps.

Amy C. Smith, DNP, RN, ACNS-BC, FACHE, is chief operating officer at Sharon Regional Health System in Sharon, Pennsylvania. Dr. Smith is a board certified clinical nurse specialist in adult health, with extensive expertise in leadership development, performance improvement, and system redesign. She is a certified Six Sigma black belt and holds a doctorate in nursing practice from Duquesne University in Pittsburgh, Pennsylvania; a master of science in nursing from Gannon University in Erie, Pennsylvania; and a bachelor of science in nursing *summa cum laude* from the University of Pittsburgh. Dr. Smith has worked in a wide variety of clinical and management roles and also maintains a private practice as a health and wellness nurse coach through her company Nurse Leader Coach LLC.

Clifford E. Brubaker, PhD, is distinguished service professor and dean emeritus of the School of Health and Rehabilitation Sciences (SHRS) at the University of

Pittsburgh. He was a professor and dean of SHRS for 24 years while also serving as a professor in the Departments of Neurological Surgery and Orthopedic Surgery of the University of Pittsburgh's School of Medicine, McGowan Institute for Regenerative Medicine, and Clinical and Translational Science Institute. Dr. Brubaker holds adjunct appointments in the Robotics Institute of the School of Computer Science at Carnegie Mellon University and in the School of Life Science and Technology at Xi'an Jiaotong University in China. Prior to joining the University of Pittsburgh, he was a professor at the University of Virginia for 18 years, with appointments in the School of Education and the Departments of Orthopedics and Biomedical Engineering in the Schools of Medicine and Engineering, respectively. Dr. Brubaker received his doctorate from the University of Oregon, where for seven years he was assistant professor of health and physical education. He has been the principal investigator and co-principal investigator for rehabilitation engineering centers at the University of Virginia and the University of Pittsburgh, working on research focused on wheelchair design and performance and seat cushion design for pressure relief. Dr. Brubaker holds six US patents and has served on review panels for the National Institutes of Health, the National Science Foundation, and the Institute of Medicine. He has led delegations to Moscow and Saint Petersburg, Russia, and hosted a reciprocal visit of engineers from Moscow's Central Machine Building Institute on behalf of the US State Department's Bureau of Human Rights and Humanitarian Affairs. Dr. Brubaker also has served as a consultant to institutions in the United States, China, and India.